INTRODUCING THERAPEUTIC ROBOTICS FOR AUTISM

INTRODUCING THERAPEUTIC ROBOTICS FOR AUTISM

BY

RAHEEL NAWAZ

Staffordshire University, UK

AND

SARA ALI

National University of Sciences and Technology (NUST), Pakistan

United Kingdom – North America – Japan – India
Malaysia – China

Emerald Publishing Limited
Howard House, Wagon Lane, Bingley BD16 1WA, UK

First edition 2023

British Library Cataloguing in Publication Data
A catalogue record for this book is available from the British Library

ISBN: 978-1-80262-778-7 (Print)
ISBN: 978-1-80262-777-0 (Online)
ISBN: 978-1-80262-779-4 (Epub)

Printed and bound by CPI Group (UK) Ltd, Croydon, CR0 4YY

ISOQAR REGISTERED
ISOQAR certified Management System, awarded to Emerald for adherence to Environmental standard ISO 14001:2004.

Certificate Number 1985
ISO 14001

INVESTOR IN PEOPLE

To Zuna, my soulmate!
(Professor Raheel Nawaz)

To Najla Ali, my mother!
(Dr Sara Ali)

CONTENTS

LIST OF ABBREVIATIONS

AAC	Augmentative and Alternative Communication
ABA	Applied Behaviour Analysis
ADL	Activities of Daily Life
ADDM	Autism and Developmental Disabilities Monitoring
ADI-R	Autism Diagnostic Interview-Revised
ADOS	Autism Diagnostic Observation Schedule
ADOS-G	Autism Diagnostic Observation Scheduled – Generic
AI	Artificial Intelligence
ASD	Autism Spectrum Disorder
ASSQ	Autism Spectrum Screening Questionnaire
AT	Assistive Technology
BCI	Brain–Computer Interface
CARS	Childhood Autism Rating Scale
CBT	Cognitive Behavioural Therapy
CDC	Centers for Disease Control and Prevention
CHAT	Checklist for Autism in Toddlers
DSM	Diagnostic and Statistical Manual of Mental Disorders
EEG	Electroencephalogram
ESDM	Early Start Denver Model
GUI	Graphical User Interface
hHRL	hierarchical Human–Robot Learning
HRI	Human–Robot Interaction
LTM	Least-to-Most
ML	Machine Learning
MMR	Measles-Mumps-Rubella
M-CHAT	Modified Checklist for Autism in Toddlers
OT	Occupational Therapy
PC	Personal Computer
PDD	Pervasive Developmental Disorder
PDD-NOS	Pervasive Developmental Disorder Not Otherwise Specified
RAAT	Robot-Assisted Autism Therapy

RAT	Robot-Assisted Therapy
SAR	Socially Assistive Robots
SCQ	Social Communication Questionnaire
SDGs	Sustainable Development Goals
SGD	Speech Generating Device
SRS	Social Responsiveness Scale
TEACCH	Treatment and Education of Autistic and Related Communication Handicapped Children
TD	Typically Developed
VR	Virtual Reality
VSD	Visual Scene Display
WOZ	Wizard of Oz
WHO	World Health Organization

ABOUT THE AUTHORS

Raheel Nawaz, PFHEA, is the Pro Vice-Chancellor (Digital Transformation) at Staffordshire University, UK. He is a renowned expert in industry-academia co-creation and is a world leading researcher in Applied Artificial Intelligence and Digital Education. He is a board member for four research and charitable organisations and regularly advises national policy organisations. He has published over 150 research articles in leading journals and conferences and has delivered keynote and invited talks at prestigious conferences and venues including European Organization for Nuclear Research (CERN), Fujitsu, Microsoft and Facebook.

Sara Ali is an Assistant Professor in Robotics and Artificial Intelligence (R&AI) Department, School of Mechanical and Manufacturing Engineering (SMME), National University of Sciences and Technology (NUST), Pakistan. Her research interests include human–robot interaction, interactive robotics, virtual reality, and human–machine interaction, controls, sensor system. She is the Principal Investigator (PI) of Human–Robot Interaction (HRI) lab at the National University of Sciences and Technology.

ACKNOWLEDGEMENTS

We would like to thank the following colleagues and friends for their valuable input in refining the manuscript.

Dr Adrian Morley
Mr Muhammad Baber Sial
Dr Muhammad Asad Bilal Fayyaz

1

INTRODUCTION TO AUTISM – UNIQUELY HUMAN

Autism Spectrum Disorder (ASD) can present significant social, communication and behavioural challenges to those who suffer from it and their carers (e.g. parents and relatives). Considering the sensitivity and significance of ASD, this work will discuss the latest techniques to improve the communication and behaviour of children using Robot-Assisted Therapies (RATs). The work will discuss autism, the prevalence of autism, state-of-the-art and impact of RATs and their associated problems. It will outline robotic interventions which can be carried out at home, making it accessible to carers without the need of a therapist. This review considers the diversity of our audience, hence, the language used is simple, terminologies explained, and practical recommendations are made for carers, therapists, psychologists, roboticists and researchers in the cognitive sciences, Artificial Intelligence (AI) and Human–Robot Interaction (HRI). Although, some work exists in the domain of RATs, scarcely any work exists discussing RAT for children with ASD, their impact, and future policies.

The first chapter of our book will discuss autism itself along with its history, assessment and use of robots for therapy. This includes outlining autism as a clinical condition, its prevalence, scales of assessment, causes and prognosis among children. Following the introduction, the impact of autism on the development and behaviour of children is discussed before connecting it to the clinical findings and therapeutic intervention. Later chapters will discuss RAT for children with ASD and its impact before concluding with some recommendations and policy proposals.

1.1. WHAT IS AUTISM?

ASD is defined as a developmental disability with recurrent deficits in social interaction and the existence of confined, repetitive patterns of behaviours, interests or activities (American Psychiatric Association & Others, 2013). Some common characteristics of ASD are avoiding eye contact, difficulties with emotional regulation or interpreting feelings, and exhibiting a limited range of activities and interests (American Psychiatric Association & Others, 1980). Other most recurring features of ASD are atypical patterns of activities and behaviours, for example, difficulty in transitioning from one activity to another, focussing on minutiae and atypical reactions to stimuli (World Health Organization (WHO), 2022). Epilepsy, depression, anxiety and attention-deficit hyperactivity disorder are some of the commonly co-occurring disorders in individuals with autism. Children with ASD can hide some of their emotional expressions while interacting. They can also miss some important signs of non-verbal communication (e.g. body language and in particular facial emotions) (Moore, 2002). Furthermore, children with autism show limited adaption to change and generalisation of learnt skills (Lahiri, 2020).

It is thought that ASD affects about 7.5 million people globally. A report from the Centers for Disease Control and Prevention (CDC) in 2020 states that around 1 in 54 children are diagnosed with ASD and lack communication skills including verbal, non-verbal and social cues. The reports mentioned that autism is four times more dominant in boys than girls across all races, ethnicities and social groups (Maenner et al., 2020). As mentioned earlier, social and communication skills are significantly affected in children with ASD, which means the condition directly affects the lifestyles of their family members. Direct family members who are carers of children with ASD can find it difficult to acquire a job that can accommodate their responsibilities, affecting their social and economic lifestyle.

Five different types of Pervasive Developmental Disorders (PDDs) are recognised: Autistic Disorder; Asperger's Disorder; Rett's Disorder; Childhood Disintegrative Disorder; and Pervasive Developmental Disorder Not Otherwise Specified (PDD-NOS). Asperger syndrome is closest to autism in terms of symptoms and causes with some differences, for example, no substantial delay in language and cognitive development (Volkmar, State, & Klin, 2009). Autism, Asperger syndrome and PDD-NOS are all referred to as ASD (American Academy of Pediatrics Council on Children With Disabilities, 2007) or autistic disorders (Freitag, 2007), whereas autism is also referred as autistic disorder, childhood autism or infantile autism. The present work will refer to 'autism' as the basic autistic disorder; nonetheless, it is essential to mention that autism, ASD, and PDD are all used interchangeably in clinical practice (Caronna, Milunsky, & Tager-Flusberg, 2008).

Autism symptoms are identified at an early age; however, it is rarely diagnosed at the initial stages. The first indication usually occurs when a child is at the age of three. Before the symptoms of autism are discussed, it is important to mention that every individual has different needs depending on the level of autism they experience. Some can live an independent life, whereas others may require lifelong care and assistance. With that acknowledgement, we shall discuss the symptoms of autism in detail.

1.1.1. Spectrum of Autism

Often the word 'spectrum' is associated with autism. This refers to the range of symptoms that children with ASD can exhibit, encompassing a wide variety of skills deficits. These varying impairments may include delayed developments, repetitive behaviour such as hand flapping and rocking, high-functioning individuals with active but distinctly odd social approaches, narrowly focussed interests, verbose and pedantic communication (Happé, 1999). Since the spectrum of behaviour is infinite, the distinction between diagnostic categories must be arbitrary (Geschwind, 2009).

1.2. HISTORY OF AUTISM

Eugen Bleuler, who was a psychiatrist, coined the term 'autism' in 1908 to characterise a schizophrenic patient who locked himself from the outside world. The word 'autism' has an interesting epistemology. Autism is derived from the Greek word 'autós,' which is defined as 'morbid self-admiration and seclusion inside oneself' (Bleuler, 1912).

Later in the 1940s, Hans Asperger and Leo Kanner were considered pioneers for their contribution to research in autism, where Kanner studied seriously affected young individuals and Asperger studied highly capable children. They researched these two extreme cases for three decades and their research and ideas are being still used by doctors (Kanner, 1943). Leo Kanner's study group consist of 11 children with the following characteristics:

- Difficulty in social life
- Difficulty in adapting to changes in routine
- Sensitivity to stimuli (especially sound)

- Food resistance and allergies
- Good intellectual potential
- Echolalia (tendency to repeat words).

Hans Asperger group had the same characteristics except the group did not have the problem of Echolalia. He, however, added to the description of these children that they differ in behaviour and motor skills. Afterwards, another psychologist Bruno Bettelheim investigated the effects of therapy sessions conducted on children with autism. He observed that children with autism all had emotionally 'cold' mothers, and later proposed this as his hypothesis. However, the hypothesis was soon rejected by Bernard Rimland, who himself had a child with autism. Autism gained more recognition in the 1970s and 1980s. The Erica Foundation started to provide counselling and education to psychotic children that included autistic children as autism was being misdiagnosed as 'mental retardation' or psychosis. Later the work of Asperger was translated into English, which gained attention among researchers. The work convinced many that it is caused by neurological disorders and other genetic illnesses such as tuberous sclerosis, metabolic disturbances such as Phenylketonuria (PKU), or chromosomal abnormalities such as fragile X syndrome, rather than by parenting. This renewed interest in the domain of autism led to many notable events since this period, including (Parents, 2022):

- In 1980, 'Infantile autism' was included as a condition in the Diagnostic and Statistical Manual of Mental Disorders (DSM) rather than under schizophrenia among children.
- In 1987, the DSM replaced 'infantile autism' with a more extensive definition of 'autism disorder' which included a checklist of diagnostic criteria.
- In 1988, the hit film 'Rain Man' was released which raised popular awareness of the condition. In it, Dustin Hoffman acted as an autistic savant with a photographic memory and an ability to calculate huge numbers in his head.
- In 1991, the US Federal Government classified 'autism' as a special category within Education, leading public schools to recognise the special treatment for children with autism.
- In 1994, Asperger's Syndrome was added to the DSM, including the individuals with high-functioning capability.
- In 1998, a study published in Lancet claimed that the measles-mumps-rubella (MMR) vaccine causes autism which was later debunked.

- In 2000, vaccine producers removed a mercury-based preservative called thimerosal from all routinely given paediatric vaccines.
- In 2009, US CDC started the estimation of autism approach which significantly helped screening and diagnostic techniques.
- In 2013, DSM-5 was presented according to which all subcategories of the condition were placed under a single umbrella diagnosis of ASD.

From 2013 onwards, experts have viewed autism as a continuous spectrum of conditions. There have been no further revisions to the DSM-5.

1.3. PREVALENCE OF AUTISM

The recognition of Autism led to many further studies and the recording of cases by medical practitioners. As a result, in the last few decades, an increasing number of autism cases have been diagnosed. In the 1960s–1970s, the initial investigation in Europe and United States suggests 2–4 cases per 1,000 children (Lotter, 1967; Rutter, 2005). This number increased drastically following the diagnostic criteria of autism in the late 1980s–1990s (Fombonne, 2009; Rice, 2013; Rutter, 2005).

The United States accepted 'ASD' in the category of those who are eligible for receiving special education, significantly increasing the number of children enrolled in the education system under this category. Often children who were misdiagnosed or classified as having an intellectual impairment were now classified as autism through a process known as 'diagnostic substitution', contributing to the rise in ASD cases among children (Maenner et al., 2014). Epidemiological studies also suggest that the development of diagnostic criteria and incorporation of the concept of autism as a spectrum of impairments during the later decades of the twentieth century can be attributed to the rise in prevalence of autism (Fombonne, 2009; King & Bearman, 2009; Rice, 2013). Other factors like increased clinician training, availability of standard screening and diagnostic tools, media awareness and outreach are also recognised as contributing to the increase in the prevalence rate.

The CDC has been tracking autism cases since 1996 and later formed the Autism and Developmental Disabilities Monitoring (ADDM) Network. Since 2010, the ADDM Network has been collecting data on ASD prevalence and its early detection among children aged 4 years. The CDC estimated that there are about 5.5 million adults with ASD in the United States (2.21% of the total population) (CDC, 2022). Data from modelling of state-based populations and parent surveys suggest a significant gender-bias, with more men affected than women [4.3 million male adults (3.62%) compared to 1.1 million female adults (0.86%)] (CDC, 2022). The prevalence trend of autism reported in the United States is based on four different data types which include:

1. Epidemiologic studies
2. Special education 'child counts'
3. Administrative data on developmental services from the state of California
4. National surveys based on parental reports.

To keep the records at national level, large-scale, nationally represented population-based epidemiologic studies should be undertaken regularly, thereby, employing verified and similar techniques and diagnostic criteria over time.

The ADDM Network tracks the prevalence of ASD at the age of eight years, since at this age they are more likely to have the disorder throughout their childhood. Since 2000, they have monitored ASD in 8-year-old children every two years in various US sites, implementing procedures that have been consistent throughout time and are based on the DSM, 4th Edition diagnostic criteria (American Psychiatric Association & Others, 2013). Furthermore, it has been established through research that the median age at which a formal diagnosis of ASD is declared is 5.2 to 5.7 years (Tribune, 2022). Pharmacological and Interventional therapies have shown promising results for ASD patients besides the traditional education and behavioural therapies. For example, a few people have improved after receiving some interventional treatment, e.g. deep brain stimulation.

Unfortunately, even after so much awareness about autism, it is considered a stigma and therefore under reported or not reported at all in some countries. For example, according to the Pakistan Autism Society, around 400,000 children in Pakistan are diagnosed with ASD. However this number is under-reported because many are reluctant to report a mental disorder (Shattuck, 2006).

1.4. PRELIMINARY ASSESSMENT AND SCREENING OF AUTISM

Initial diagnostics are often done by the parents or carers of children with ASD. About half of the parents are reported to be aware of their child's atypical behaviour when their child is only 18 months and about 4/5th are aware of this behaviour when the child is about 24 months. The usual atypical behaviour among children includes missing the milestone, such as

- no response to their name by the age of 6 months
- no eye-to-eye gaze contact

- absence of babbling by the age of 12 months
- lack of gestures
- non-appearance of a single word by age of 16 months
- no phrases (2 words or more) by the age of 24 months
- lack of general social and language skills.

Failure to achieve any of these milestones is a key indicator of potential ASD and parents should proceed with further evaluation of autism. By the age of 18 months, half of the parents of children with ASD are aware of their child's atypical behaviours, and about four-fifths are aware by the age of 24 months (Landa, 2008). The usual behaviour of a child includes missing the milestone; no response to the name by the age of 6 months, no eye-to-eye gaze contact, absence of babbling by the age of 12 months, no gestures, non-appearance of a single word by age of 16 months or no phrases (2 words) by the age of 24 months, lack of social and language skills. Failure to achieve any of the mentioned milestones is the key indicator that parents should proceed with further evaluation for autism. A delay in evaluation or non-early diagnosis can have long-term effects. The trend for screening the child for autism varies in different parts of the world. For example, in Japan, the screening of all children is done at 18 and 24 months whereas in the UK only children whose parents or doctors find early signs of autism are screened.

There are different screening tools available for rating autism. The Checklist for Autism in Toddlers (CHAT), Modified Checklist for Autism in Toddlers (M-CHAT) and the Early Screening of Autistic Traits Questionnaire are a few of the early screening tools available (Landa, 2008). However, these tools do not distinguish autism from other developmental disorders. For this purpose, wideband screening tools should be used that may or may not include genetic screening, depending upon the case (Lintas & Persico, 2009).

1.5. SCALES FOR AUTISM ASSESSMENT

As outlined, Autism can be characterised by the difficulty in forming social bonds, maintaining social contact and atypical interest profile. This behaviour leads to the use of repetitive language, which results in delayed language acquisition and development of language (Dumont-Mathieu & Fein, 2005). This restricted children's ability to imitate and participate in play after having stereotyped body movements and usual association with objects (American Psychiatric Association & Others, 2013). Even though the mentioned characteristics are usually obvious to observers, there remains a need for quantifiable measures through which assessments of the disorder's severity can be obtained. To achieve a quantifiable measure, different scales and measures are available, e.g. Childhood Autism Rating Scale (CARS), Social Responsiveness Scale (SRS), Autism Diagnostic Observation Scheduled – Generic (ADOS-G), Autism Diagnostic Interview-Revised (ADI-R), and Social Communication Questionnaire (SCQ).

The scales are designed to obtain detailed feedback from either carers or parents, which is then used to quantify the level of severity of the autism. For example, the SRS scale is based on 65 questions in the form of a questionnaire, where each response is ranged from 'Not True' to 'Almost Always True'. The given questionnaire is filled by carers or parents of children between the age group of 4 and 8 years (Constantino et al., 2003). This test has strong psychometric qualities and cross-cultural validity in the assessment of autism, helping to quantify the severity of autism-related symptoms (Rutter, Bailey, & Lord, 2003).

The SCQ test is similar to SRS and has 40 questions. The questions required binary responses from parents and carers who have detailed information about their children's developmental behaviour. The available versions of SCQ are 'Current' and 'Lifetime'. The SCQ score can be used to discriminate ASD from non-ASD individuals (Rutter, Bailey, et al., 2003). The ADI-R scale consists of 93 items through input from caregivers in the form of a semi-structured interview. The scale can be applied to individuals with a mental age above 18 months. Some questions in SCQ are adapted from ADI (Lord et al., 1997).The most simple and relevant scale is CARS, which was developed by Schopler, Reichler, and Renner (1988). It consists of a 15-item questionnaire, which uses a 4-point Likert scale to score the behaviour of an individual ranging from 1, which represents no evidence of autism, to 4, which represents severe autism. This is generally used for children above 2 years. The 14 categories within this test deal with the behaviour associated with autism, while the 15th category is used to rate the general symptoms of autism in the individual (Chlebowski, Green, Barton, & Fein, 2010).

Another important scale is the high-functioning Autism Spectrum Screening Questionnaire (ASSQ), which consists of 27 items used for evaluating symptoms that distinguish between Asperger syndrome and other high-functioning ASDs. The questionnaire uses a 3-point rating scale, where 0 is used to denote 'normalcy', 1 for 'abnormality' and 2 for 'substantial abnormality'. The awarded score from this scale can be between 0 and 54. The scale, however, does not work with the individuals with low-functioning autism, i.e. the ones with moderate-severe mental retardation. An updated, extended version of ASSQ (ASSQ-REV) also exists particularly for screening the female phenotype of ASD (Kopp & Gillberg, 2011).

Once the autistic feature and severity of an individual has been determined using these scales, the next step for the family is to seek out the intervention that will best meet the child's unique needs depending on the type of challenge he/she possesses.

1.6. CAUSES AND PROGNOSIS OF AUTISM

Autism's unique trifecta of symptoms has long been assumed to have a single origin at the genetic, cognitive, and neurological levels (Happé & Ronald, 2008). However, there is growing evidence that autism is a multifaceted disorder with multiple origins that frequently co-occur (Happé, Ronald, & Plomin, 2006). Autism has a significant genetic basis, yet the genetics of autism are complex, and it is uncertain which combination is more responsible for its cause; uncommon mutations with substantial effects or uncommon multigene combinations of common genetic variants (Abrahams & Geschwind, 2008; Buxbaum, 2009). Through mapping the genomes of autistic people and their parents, many genes have been linked to autism (Sanders et al., 2015). Moreover, the foetus's neurodevelopment is influenced by maternal diet and inflammation during preconception and pregnancy. Intrauterine growth restriction (both term and preterm new borns) is also linked to autism (Vohr, Davis, Wanke, & Krebs, 2017). Air pollution, particularly heavy metals and particles may raise the incidence of autism during pregnancy (Lam et al., 2016; Lyall, Schmidt, & Hertz-Picciotto, 2014). Certain foods, infectious diseases, solvents, phthalates, and phenols used in plastic products, pesticides, brominated flame retardants, alcohol, smoking, illicit substances, immunisations, and prenatal stress have all been claimed (without definitive proof) to contribute to or exacerbate autism (Newschaffer et al., 2007).

Some changes during the development of the brain have also been linked to autism symptoms. However, the exact cause of autism is still unknown. In this regard, researchers claim that the mechanism of autism can be divided into two main areas:

1. Pathophysiology of brain structures and processes linked to autism
2. Neuropsychological links between brain structures and behaviours (London, 2007).

Another reported cause of autism is gut-brain axis abnormalities (Israelyan & Margolis, 2019; Rao & Gershon, 2016; Wasilewska & Klukowski, 2015). In 2015, researchers concluded that neuroinflammation and dysfunction of the brain are due to immune dysregulation, gastrointestinal inflammation, malfunction of the autonomic nervous system, gut flora alterations, and food metabolites (Wasilewska & Klukowski, 2015). Another analysis report in 2016 suggests that the anomalies in the enteric nervous system might have a role in neurological disorders including autism. The immune system and neural connections may be a conduit for diseases which starts in the intestine and travel to the brain (Rao & Gershon, 2016).

Currently, there is no known cure of autism and regardless of the cause of autism, the aim when treating an autistic child is to reduce the related deficits and family distress. Treatment predominantly aims to improve quality of life and functional independence (Levy, Mandell, & Schultz, 2009). In some cases, treatment may reduce the severity of symptoms to such an extent that a patient may lose their ASD diagnostic traits (Levy et al., 2009). Though the core deficiencies persist in an autistic person, however, symptoms are less severe as age progresses (Rapin & Tuchman, 2008). However, very little research and high-quality analysis of long-term prognosis has been done, which makes it harder to analyse the situation in middle age groups (Seltzer, Shattuck, Abbeduto, & Greenberg, 2004).

1.7. MANAGING AUTISM

Due to the stigma and psychosocial variables, autistic people are likely to be exposed to greater stress levels, which may lead to more severity of their autism and other mental health problems (Botha & Frost, 2020). Besides social stigma and obstacles in transitioning to adulthood, the job opportunities for people with autism are very few (Hendricks & Wehman, 2009). To ensure a healthy lifestyle with better job opportunities in society, a proper management is required through education, clinical therapies, medication or robotic interventions. Treatments and interventions are tailored according to the demands of autistic children, but generally the responsiveness from therapy and better outcomes are associated with children with higher IQs (Smith & Iadarola, 2015).

The family and education system is primarily responsible for caring for or managing children with autism (Levy et al., 2009). The education system typically works through 'behavioural analysts' such as special education teachers, speech pathologists and licenced psychologists (Ospina et al., 2008). In terms of interventions, methodological flaws in intervention studies limit conclusive findings on efficacy (Ospina et al., 2008). This might be because every child with autism has a different degree of issues with social interaction, empathy, communication, and flexible behaviour. However, in recent years, the development of robotic interventions (Ali, et al., 2019) and evidence-based therapies have progressed (Smith & Iadarola, 2015) in which adaptive therapies are being considered. These therapies adapt themselves according to the child's needs and behaviour. Although it is better to have some treatment rather than none, the methodological quality of systematic reviews of these studies is improving with time.

Intensive long-term special education programmes and behaviour therapy are targeted among children to help them develop self-care, communication and employment skills along with enhancing functioning, reducing symptom severity and maladaptive behaviours (American Academy of Pediatrics Council on Children With Disabilities, 2007; Howlin, Magiati, & Charman, 2009). Drugs can be used to treat related symptoms such as irritation, inattention, or repetitive behaviour patterns but no research provides evidence where drugs are used to cure core symptoms (Ji & Findling, 2015). Educational Interventions are common interventions that focus on Applied Behaviour Analysis (ABA), developmental models, structured teaching, speech and language therapy, social skills therapy and occupational therapy (OT) (Smith & Iadarola, 2015). ABA therapy has been shown to improve communication and adaptive functioning in pre-schoolers with autism as well as for boosting the intellectual performance of the child (American Academy of Pediatrics Council on Children With Disabilities, 2007; Eikeseth, 2009). Moreover, teachers implementing interventions in a more naturalistic form of ABA combined with a developmental social pragmatic approach has proven to show improvement in communication skills of children with ASD. Alongside these interventions and therapies, some debate among educators and academics is undergoing on the inclusiveness of autistic children in the general schooling group (Simpson, de Boer-Ott, & Smith-Myles, 2003).

1.8. AUTISM AND ROBOTS

Robots from the domain of Socially Assistive Robots (SAR) are increasingly being used to treat autistic children and improve their social interaction skills (Scassellati, Admoni, & Matarić, 2012). Technological advancement in socially assistive robots has launched a promising new method for individuals with autism to get more tailored care according to their needs in recent years. In principle, these robots can assist human therapists and take over more monotonous training routines. The use of AI may also allow for a more personalised experience (MIT Technology Review, 2022). Independently, Robots are currently unable to identify and respond to behavioural stimuli, especially in atypical users and real-world settings. Therefore, researchers have implemented AI and machine learning (ML) algorithms to build adaptive therapies in which robot can monitor participants' engagement and the child's interest in the intervention (EurekAlert, 2022). Due to unavailability and affordability issues of human therapists, RATs are becoming popular among care providers.

Following our discussion on Autism, its history and prevalence along with its diagnosis and the use of robots for its therapies, Chapter 2 will discuss evolving research field for therapeutic interventions using RATs. It discusses some conventional robotic interventions which can improve the communications skills of children with ASD and highlights some main projects on this subject including DREAM and AURORA, etc. This will separately present the robotic intervention for each focussed impairment such as joint attention, verbal and non-verbal communication skills, interventions for imitation, interventions based on physical play skills, game-based interventions and interventions based on electroencephalogram (EEG) signals. Moreover, this chapter will compare the advantages and disadvantages of different robotic therapeutic investigations done so far, including the comparison of various factors such as accuracy, improvement, body-worn sensors (if used), type and number of robots. Finally, it will discuss the critical need to make these therapies effective, considering the increasing number of children with ASD and the objective to provide a better quality of life.

Chapter 3 will investigate the impact of various robotic therapies. This chapter will introduce and summarise the efficiency and impact of robotic interventions done so far, including sociopsychological and physiological effects of RAT for children with autism. This will compare various important factors that affect the improvement in communication skills of ASD children including the factors for adherence and acceptability of robotic intervention by a child. Furthermore, it will discuss the impact of robot therapeutic intervention on families of children with ASD including the impact on learning opportunities, and the overall effectiveness of social robots in teaching. The chapter will evaluate the impact by assessing the attention, engagement, anxiety, and disruptive and repetitive behaviour of children with autism. This chapter will aim to present the impact of therapies so that it will help design the future intervention techniques for improving the communication skills (verbal and non-verbal), joint attention, imitation and behavioural aspects including the impact of cultural difference in children's interaction with robots, and how it could affect their distrust. The most important by-product of this chapter will be closer interaction among different therapeutic techniques for designing a better-assisted intervention.

Finally, the last chapter will focus on suggesting the future direction including policy recommendations for RATs in the light of the literature presented above. The policies and future directions will be focussed on interdisciplinary research approaches; therefore, it will be beneficial for all cross-disciplinary domains aiming to develop robotic interventions in future. The focus will be on discussing the issues related to accessibility, affordability and the administrative burden regarding robotic interventions. Appropriate policies for robust robotic therapies that can increase engagement while keeping in view the ease and accessibility are proposed. While suggesting future directions and policies, interaction, safety, autonomy, modularity, acceptability by both parents and child and adaptability will be kept in regard. This chapter will also shed light on the direction of future research, which addresses whether social learning from robots can be generalised to a universal case.

2

MACHINES AND AUTISM

Robots as assistive technology (AT) is the fastest-growing field for the therapy of children with autism. This chapter delves into the use of robots in therapies for helping children with autism to develop social and communication skills. Research in robotics proposes that robots can therapeutically help because children with ASD are more inclined towards robots rather than humans, and this concept is supported by autism experts as children with autism have a predilection for things over other persons and robots are considered as toys by children. This chapter will explore how different robotic therapies are affecting the social and communication skills in children with ASD using robots, while focussing on specific interventions for certain impairments. RATs are models of human–robot relationship developed for a broader society where robots can take on the role of the therapist in an interactive encounter.

2.1. AUTISM AND TECHNOLOGY

As children with autism are considered to exhibit something between social and asocial behaviour, the role of robots in therapeutic interventions for children with autism can be considered between humans and machines. These robots can be considered as exhibiting human traits without a layer of complexity that can act as a barrier to communication with children with ASD, leading to greater comfort and responsiveness. The use of robotics in therapy provokes many pertinent questions for both users and researchers, for example:

1. Can anthropomorphic robots act social enough to develop social interaction and communication skills in children with ASD?
2. What does social interaction mean for those individuals for whom basic interaction can be bewildering and difficult?

3. Can machines play the role of intermediaries intended to therapeutically help children with autism?

In the early twenty-first century, we are on the verge of a new technologically mediated sociality, where robots are not only used for therapeutic intervention but also to support several physical disabilities. Considering the wide range of impairments on the autism spectrum, an appropriate way of using machines should include an adaptation of therapy according to the child's need to maximise the benefits of assisted therapies. As individuals with autism are prescribed different types of medicines, similarly, the therapeutic session with Robots for each autistic person can be customised accordingly (Shukla et al., 2015). Therefore the controllable autonomy of the robot is a basic requirement for a robot to be an acceptable social partner (Adams & Robinson, 2011). Children who are not willing to co-operate with the therapist have shown promising results when interacting with robots. Children can prefer robots over human therapists because of the predictive nature of robots that builds a high degree of motivation and engagement in the individual (Rabbitt, Kazdin, & Scassellati, 2015). Therefore, using robots as mediators between a human therapist and a child with autism can have beneficial results (Esteban et al., 2017). Socially Assistive Robots (SARs) are more helpful for individuals with in-person communication disabilities as communicating with robots can be less menacing than with a human (Alemi, Meghdari, Basiri, & Taheri, 2015; Kozima, Nakagawa, & Yasuda, 2005).

2.2. INTERVENTION STRATEGIES

An important aspect for any kind of intervention for children with ASD is to motivate and reward the social behaviour of the child (Kasari, Freeman, & Paparella, 2006). Several methods of intervention are available depending upon the child's impairment and requirement. Treatments include social stories, verbal and non-verbal social skills training, interactions with typical peers, Cognitive Behavioural Therapy (CBT) and computer face processing games (Bauminger, 2002; Carter et al., 2004; Chiang, Lee, Frey, & McCormick, 2004; Nakabayashi & Matsumoto, 2003). Experimentation and research have explored the effectiveness of a humanoid robot for helping children with autism. Evidence suggests a high degree of impact, keeping in view the opinion of autism experts (including psychiatrists, educationalists and roboticists). Some other therapies include parental education and training, social skills training and speech-language therapy, ABA, sensory integration/OT, medication, Early Start Denver Model (ESDM) Therapy, Treatment and

Education of Autistic and Related Communication Handicapped Children (TEACCH). This chapter will focus on ABA as it is the most common implemented intervention.

2.2.1. Applied Behaviour Analysis

ABA is the most well-known intervention for improvement in the behaviour of children with ASD (Rosenwasser & Axelrod, 2001). ABA is founded on the idea that most social behaviours are learnt over time because of interactions between the individual and his/her environment, and that environmental cues and stimuli can impact how a person with ASD acts (Mace, 1994). ABA therapies include cognition and speech-language development for children with ASD. ABA is a stepwise and highly structured learning process followed by a reward. The following are some of the most well-known studies on ABA therapies:

1. Lovaas provided intense ABA therapy to 19 children for 40 hours each week over two years. With minimal support, 9 out of 19 children did better in school, while 1 out of every 40 children in the control group improved significantly (Lovaas, 1987).
2. Landa and Kalb used ABA on 48 children aged 2 to 6 years for 6 months and saw significant improvements in IQ, social skills and autism alleviation (Landa & Kalb, 2012).
3. Cohen et al. compared 21 children who received 35–40 hours of ABA therapy per week to 21 children who were in the control group. After 3 years, 17 out of 21 children who received ABA therapy were fully integrated into normal education with no or limited support, whereas only 1out of every 21 children in the control group were fully integrated into regular education (Cohen, Amerine-Dickens, & Smith, 2006).

The success rate of ABA is because these therapeutic methods are scientifically supported and based on behavioural analysis research, which covers the study of human behaviour and the influence of environmental conditions in children with ASD. ABA therapies for behavioural analysis use concepts and strategies to reinforce positive behaviours and support the development of new communication skills in children with ASD. One of the main reasons for successful ABA strategies is positive reinforcement, where an improved behaviour followed by some reward is likely to progress at a higher rate. This concept of positive reinforcement is the key to developing positive behaviour change over time, once the therapist has identified a certain goal to reach in behaviour. Another concept of analysis is Antecedent, Behaviour and Consequence. It is an important three-step process that helps us to teach and understand the behaviour of children with autism, where antecedents occur before the behaviour and consequences occur after the behaviour. As such, it is a crucial part to understand the ABA program.

In summary, the development of social robots for children with autism has marked a turning point in autism studies. Mechanical metaphors of autism proliferate in the psychiatric and robot therapy literature asserting repeatedly that there is a special affinity between children with autism and robots. Studies have shown promising results that demonstrate improvement in main core impairment and child's behaviour through robotic therapeutic interventions (Breazeal, 2009; Dautenhahn & Werry, 2004; Peca et al., 2016; Robins, Dautenhahn, Te Boekhorst, & Billard, 2005; Scassellati, 2005; Thill, Pop, Belpaeme, Ziemke, & Vanderborght, 2012). Robotic therapies are also gaining attention due to their controllability, accuracy and predictability (Feng, Jia, Chen, & Li, 2016). There are many kinds of robots available for robotic therapeutic interventions for children with ASD. It includes a variety of embodiments including anthropomorphic as well as zoomorphic (animal-like) robots. Studies have shown that there is an effect of embodiment or robotic platform on the behaviour of ASD children. The effect of the robotic platform on the therapy is discussed in detail in the following section.

2.3. AUGMENTATIVE AND ALTERNATIVE COMMUNICATION FOR CHILDREN WITH AUTISM

Augmentative and Alternative Communication (AAC) is an intensive and promising treatment approach to address communication needs using current technology. However, it can be difficult to convince practicing clinicians about the efficacy of AAC in terms of language and communication development. This section aims to aid the reader's understanding of the potential for AAC by providing background knowledge about different types of AAC. The American Speech-Language Hearing Association defines any form of communication other than oral communication that expresses thoughts, needs, wants and ideas as a type of AAC (ASHA, 2022). Two primary forms of AAC used for communication disorders are aided and un-aided AAC (Cardon, 2016). The main difference between two categories is that for un-aided AAC, the individual uses his/her body to convey the message such as through gestures and sign language, without using any additional equipment to facilitate the non-verbal communication. In aided AAC, additional adaptive tools are used to convey messages. The most effective for children with ASD is aided AAC that uses visual support in the form of pictures and videos, etc.

A national standards report published by the National Autism Centre is considered as a standard among research scientists and specialists in this field (Phase 2, 2015). This document declares AAC as one of the most effective emerging treatments for children with ASD at any point on the spectrum. The current research available on AAC and autism is limited due to small sample sizes and the heterogeneity of samples, however, when paired with intensive interventions remarkable results can be seen in terms of expressive language and functional communication (Dawson et al., 2010). Within AAC, there are several options, ranging from low-tech to high-tech. Low-tech options are considered best to start with and address initial behaviour issues. These include the use of 'Big Mac' buttons that initiate a question or comment, picture boards, and the use of the Picture Exchange Communication System (PECS) (Frost & Bondy, 2002). To describe the capability of AAC, the options available for high-tech devices includes fixed display, dynamic display, Visual Scene Display (VSD) and Speech Generating Devices (SGDs) (Cardon, 2016). In a fixed display option, symbols and messages remain static along with the fixed positioning of pictures on the screen. This is helpful in terms of self-corrections against mishits due to a lack of, or limited, navigation challenges on the screen. This is therefore considered best in the early process of teaching. Moreover, because of the predictability of items on screen, this is considered fairly easy to use as it demands less cognitive load while expressing the needs for communication.

In contrast, the dynamic mode extends a lot of flexibility in terms of advanced language system features that improve skills for children with ASD. This includes change in the display of screen such as opening a new screen when an option is selected. Because of such features it demands high brain cognition in response to the changing screen environment. This approach is recommended for children with better receptive language ability and a need for more complex language use. Regardless of the options selected (i.e. fixed display, dynamic display, or VSD options) all can be found in SGDs that provide voice output when the child selects a picture or a symbol for communication. For the children who already have verbal ability, SGD may encourage an increase in social initiations and decrease in communication breakdowns with unfamiliar communication partners (Wilkinson, Light, & Drager, 2012).

With the rapidly changing technology, new approaches for AAC are anticipated that include high-tech devices to treat the impairments of children with ASD. This will also include software applications, constituting an emerging area within the field of augmentative alternative communication and AT for improvement in visual attention and eye tracking (Cardon, 2016). In this regard, some of the high-tech therapies to address the impairments are discussed in this chapter.

2.4. TECHNOLOGICAL ASSISTED INTERVENTIONS AND ITS IMPLICATIONS

With the advent of new technology, the use of Personal Computers (PCs) in this field has risen in popularity due to their portability and inexpensiveness compared to AAC technology. This has opened a completely new world for developers who are now offering products to consumers not only for face-to-face interaction but also for other purposes which aid participation from their homes, schools, work, or any other environment. Similarly, mobiles phones and other personal computing devices are now a part of everyday life. This has extended potential access for learners as service providers can develop educational and behavioural services to individuals with autism using this technology. Devices such as mobile phones, tablets and touch screens computing devices have become universally available at low cost and user-friendly applications. As technology becomes a more persistent element of children's life, it has implications for both education and communication.

The most effective use of technology varies from child to child. It is not necessary that every child with ASD will learn communication from technological devices such as iDevices, etc. All these technologies, interventions and devices work for certain people in a certain way. For example, the use of mobile phone is not limited to entertainment anymore but can also be used for teaching such as ABA therapies, reinforcement learning, verbal and non-verbal communication and many other application-based therapeutic interventions for children with ASD. Multiple devices are used for therapeutic interventions for children with ASD that might include accessories to measure gaze tracking, body movement, speech, head movements, etc.

Touch screens and user-friendly Graphical User Interface (GUI) make portable devices such as tablets and phones particularly useful for individuals with ASD. Moreover, the adaptability with such devices is quicker. For example, in a case in which an individual gets irritated by loud voices, this can be handled easily by lowering the volume of device. Similarly, if the individual with ASD has problem in writing, motor skills can be improved, and frustration decreased by using the text to speech feature and touch pads for writing. Non-verbal communication is another factor that can be addressed using technology. Children who cannot communicate using verbal speech find it easier to use written words associated with pictures. In such cases, technology is being used as voice output device for these individuals (Cardon, 2016). The ability to use visual and speech inputs simultaneously can also be enhanced using technology. Moreover, technology can offer therapies that are adaptive and based on Least-to-Most (LTM) order (Ali et al., 2020). These devices also have an advantage of monitoring the performance of individual as they progress in the therapies. These devices collect data for individual's performance that can be assessed, checking for various research aspects such as dominance of brain hemisphere in visual space while doing a certain task (Mehmood, Ayaz, Ali, De Cassia Amadeu, & Sadia, 2019), categorisation of autism level using different ML algorithms (Ali et al., 2022), etc.

The speed at which technology is growing is unprecedented. Future developments may take forms that we cannot anticipate. Although apps are no newer for offering therapies to children with autism, they are now moving towards adaptability according to the child's individual need and requirements after doing visual processing and recording the feedback. They can also integrate progress evaluation for the child involved in a certain therapy. Now-a-days research is heading towards the greater and more sophisticated use of the robots in therapeutic interventions. It is believed that robots will be able to improve impairments including communication skills (verbal and non-verbal), imitation, joint attention, etc., allowing the child and their carers to focus on targeted therapies.

2.5. ARTIFICIAL HUMANS TREATING AUTISM

Machines make sense to an extent that should not be under-estimated when integrated with AI and ML algorithms, particularly focussing on humanoid robots (robots that look like humans) for treating the children with autism. There is a field dedicated to exploring the interactions between humans and machines called HRI. The reason for using robots for HRI interventions is because children with autism feel more inclined towards robots, machines and devices. Another rationale presented in the studies for why to use robots for treating autism is that as individuals with autism are mostly non-empathetic thereby, they are more attracted towards devices and machines rather than humans (Richardson, 2018). For this purpose, there are different therapies including use of wearable devices, apps and robot-assisted therapeutic interventions for children with autism. All these are focussed on developing interventions for improvement in aspects such as joint attention, imitation, verbal and non-verbal communication, etc. These interventions are discussed in this chapter individually.

2.5.1. Apps

The use of mobile phone apps is not a new concept for improving impairments in children with ASD. These apps are growing over the time, adding features of adaptability according to the child's requirement. Moreover, the apps are now developing with the feature of analysing the progress of individual over the time. AI-based algorithms can also predict child's behaviour over for future.

2.5.2. Wearables

Among various other technological interventions, one of the most interesting solutions was Google Glass released in May 2014. The expansion of companies making wearable products has increased rapidly. These glasses display information in front of the wearer's eyes, thereby putting them on the viewed image of reality in real-time. Google Glass also provides the user with applications specially built to identify the facial expressions and emotions of individuals with ASD. Researchers are also working towards creating a feasible environment for communicating with individuals with ASD by using these glasses. This will be done by giving an alert to the other user by extracting the emotion of ASD child from his/her facial expressions (The Guardian, 2022). Researchers are working on tracking the emotion and linking it with facial expressions using Google Glass. Moreover, research investigating how to teach emotion recognition and encourage increased eye contact using this wearable device is also in progress. Another technology in this category is the use of smart watch for individuals with ASD. Linked with smartphones, these devices provide additional information that can be translated in functional skill of the child. Moreover, reminders, alarms, appointments, etc., will be on the wrist of the individual making it easier for them to remember and conduct daily tasks. Similarly other wearable devices to monitor the progress of children include EEG headsets, tracking devices to monitor heart rate, movement, sleep and sweat levels.

2.5.3. Robot-Assisted Therapies

Despite some benefits of using animals for therapy, they still pose several drawbacks. They are generally difficult to control, have unpredictability in behaviour even when well-trained, and may transmit infections or provoke allergies. As a result, using robots is considered to be more appealing since they maintain the communication simplicity of animals while overcoming some of their drawbacks. As outlined in previous chapters, RAT can be used as a complementary therapy for children with ASD, and it has the potential to reduce the workload of the therapist (and thus the therapy's cost), as well as improve the social skills of these children, allowing them to function in society. Robot-Assisted Autism Therapy (RAAT) proves its effectiveness in several aspects of communication behaviour such as attention and imitation (Kim et al., 2013), identifying and understanding emotions (Zhang, Song, Tan, Wang, et al., 2019; Zhang, Song, Tan, Zhu, et al., 2019) and improving sensitivity to physical contact (Bharatharaj, Huang, Al-Jumaily, Elara, & Krägeloh, 2017; Chernyak & Gary, 2016). Given the current rate of technological advancement, there is a lot of room for innovation in treatment procedures for children with ASD, where robots have been widely used for technological interventions of children with ASD. Currently, the approach used for robotic intervention uses the Wizard of Oz (WOZ) method, where a robot is remotely controlled by a human operator to perform a certain task (Wilson & Rosenberg, 1988). However, for a consistent therapeutic intervention, the algorithm should be adaptive in order to reduce the burden on the child and therapist. RAAT are used for addressing several different issues for children with ASD such as learning social behaviours and emotions using robots, improvement in non-verbal speech gestures, enhancing the anthropomorphic thinking of children with ASD, learning complex and social rules, and relationships and contact learning, etc. (Szymona et al., 2021). RAAT is designed and focussed according on the need for impairment of the ASD child. We have discussed some of the famous RAAT to give the reader an idea about how the RAAT works.

At present, the research on RAAT usually focusses on robots' control architectures for autism intervention that controls robots without implementing the traditional methods of intervention for children with ASD. A similar architecture called B^{3}IA was proposed by Feil-Seifer and Mataric based on the control architecture of the robot (Feil-Seifer & Mataric, 2008a). The B^{3}IA architecture is composed of different modules such as the sensor and interpretation module, activity history module, behaviour network and effector module. In other research by Marino et al. (2020) the robot provides participants with emotional enhancement by giving certain hints and therefore acting as a co-therapist in this study. Pre- and post-intervention assessments show improved contextual recognition as well as an understanding of emotions using social robots. In a study by Valadão et al. (2016), the experiment was divided into three different phases, carrying the concept of complex experiments with a simple design. In phase one, the social skills of ASD subjects were accessed, in the second phase, touch and imitation were assessed and finally, in the third phase, game development skills were incorporated in which a robot was used as a mediator producing satisfactory results of this research. In another research by a Japanese specialist Kumazaki (Szymona et al., 2021), two CommU robots were used to study social functioning based on the ADOS-2 (Autism Diagnostic Observation Schedule) with robots improvising three different scenarios. This study is an assessment scale for the social functioning of patients with the SRS.

2.5.3.1. Robotic Interventions for Verbal and Non-Verbal Speech

Different therapies have been developed that focus on improvement in structured behaviour approach for non-verbal speech and gestures. The result of those therapies shows that children have improved sense of gestures and words after the treatment sessions (Buffington, Krantz, McClannahan, & Poulson, 1998). Similarly, in another study by So et al. (2016) and So, Wong, Lui, and Yip (2015), a humanoid robot NAO was used for imitating different gestures to understand non-verbal speech. Another important factor when it comes to non-verbal speech therapies is touch, which is an important developmental factor for a child as it shows a child's stable expression of positive feelings (Bai, Repetti, & Sperling, 2016). Research shows that young children who are deprived of social touch by their parents or who avoided touch develop a higher probability of sensory processing disorders such as being over-sensitive (Wilbarger, Gunnar, Schneider, & Pollak, 2010). Therefore, avoidance of social touch in the early years can be a forecaster of ASD in children (Mammen et al., 2015). This has been backed up by research which shows children with ASD react abnormally to the touch (Cascio, Gu, Schauder, Key, & Yoder, 2015; Cascio, Lorenzi, & Baranek, 2016) which in turn supports the basic clinical symptoms of ASD (Pryweller et al., 2014). RAAT have helped a lot in developing the sense of touch in children with ASD (Bauminger, 2002; Kasari et al., 2006; Kozima et al., 2005). Studies that used the social robot to teach children complex social rules showed a greater confidence in children with anthropomorphic thinking towards the robot (Carter et al., 2004). Studies have been conducted in which a robot is used to teach complex social skills to ASD children such as distrust and cheating during the sessions (Chiang et al., 2004). However, it was noted in the study that children with ASD find it difficult in learning distrust and cheating as compared to the typically developed (TD) children. This is because inhibition control is found in children with ASD, which can cause complications in ascribing mental social states. Similarly, an intervention for improving the verbal communication skills of children with ASD was performed by introducing an anthropomorphic robot, RoboParrot. RoboParrot is a parrot looking robot used to teach turn-taking skills to children with ASD. The result of the intervention showed children were more cooperative with the therapist when a robot was introduced to the interventions (Nakabayashi & Matsumoto, 2003).

Robots are also used to teach relationships and contact learning to children with ASD. For this purpose, one of the famous robots Romibo is a plush blue robot used for encouraging contact in children with autism. Such contact should not replace a conversation with parents or therapists; however, it can be a friendly companion for children.

2.5.3.2. Virtual Reality and Autism

The drawbacks of conventional therapy can be avoided by adopting latest technological approaches used for the treatment of autism. These technological interventions include both robotic and computer-based technology that can accommodate additional factors such as better communication skills, identifying and quantifying the emotions of an ASD child more technically, etc. (Yang & Zhang, 2021). Virtual reality (VR)-related technological interventions are also better in terms of controllability, personalisation and scalability of the intervention for any child with ASD according to its need. However, although for robot-based interventions, children with ASD are more inclined, the cost factor is relatively high compared with computer-based interaction. Computer-based interactions are more appropriate for generalisation, but care must be taken to avoid alienating patients from reality. For this reason, one of the best ways to relate robotic and computer based technological interventions is using VR-based therapies for autism.

Traditional teaching methods are never effective for children with ASD (Rosenwasser & Axelrod, 2001). VR is considered one of the effective modes of teaching not only for children with ASD but also for TD children as it adds a sense of reality while learning (Mace, 1994). Playing the games in VR also inculcates a sense of perception and reality, where studies show that VR improves the development of children with autism and in general. This is done using purpose-based VR interventions such as car simulation, toilet training, music simulation, etc. (Breazeal, 2009; Cohen et al., 2006; Landa & Kalb, 2012; Lovaas, 1987). All VR-related technological interventions for children with autism improve the movement of eyes by using game-based scenarios (Dautenhahn & Werry, 2004) which is helpful in the development of joint attention using motion capture technology. All these therapies use various technological means for their development such as monocular display, tracking technologies and Augmented Reality (AR) to integrate the virtual and real world together. This can be done using a video based task in a virtual environment that uses multi-sensors (Yang & Zhang, 2021). These technological elements help children with ASD due to unique advantages compared with conventional therapies. For example, patients can have the confidence that they can learn at their own pace without the pressure of judgement. Although, the development of technological interventions has extensively promoted the diagnosis, intervention and treatment of ASD, the effectiveness of therapies depends highly on the design of interventions. Moreover, to better tap the potential of an ASD child, the effectiveness of VR-based scenes for various applications are also dependent on graphical user interfaces (GUIs) of stimuli, the adaptiveness of intervention, and the avatars of virtual characters used in scenes. Studies have been done to compare the effectiveness of VR technology over other technological interventions. According to a systematic review (Mesa-Gresa, Gil-Gómez, Lozano-Quilis, & Gil-Gómez, 2018), the majority of studies only examine how participants with ASD improve after receiving VR intervention without conducting enough comparisons with either the subjects in the control group or the outcomes of other intervention techniques such as video modelling (Fitzgerald et al., 2018). Moreover, which category of autism will be the beneficiary of VR-based interventions is still a question. As VR is becoming new hotspot for future direction, therefore, this book overemphasises the technology's usefulness of VR rather than presenting the rational analysis of VR's benefits and drawbacks.

2.5.3.3. Robotic Therapy for Joint Attention and Imitation

There are few existing approaches to robot therapies that use the adaptive algorithm for improving the communication skills of children with ASD particularly focussing on joint attention. One such recent approach is Multi-Robot Interactive System (MRIS) in which the algorithm adapts itself from LTM in order to observe the child's progress in the intervention (Wasilewska & Klukowski, 2015). There are two adaptive modules, one for joint attention and the other one for imitation skills of the child with ASD. The study shows that the imitation of meaningful gestures for children with ASD is better than meaningless gestures (Eikeseth, 2009), and it addresses dominance in the visual space of ASD children using a multi-robot joint attention integrated distributed system (Rao & Gershon, 2016). In another research on robot-based therapies, the effect of different stimuli by the robot is studied to observe which stimulus works best for robotic interventions (Levy et al., 2009). Joint attention is one of the main core impairments as the transfer of eye gaze is necessary for effective communication. Children with autism lag in the ability of joint attention which is one of the major indications of autism at an early age (Peca et al., 2016). This has been addressed by different interventions that introduce robots to improve the joint attention of ASD children (Robins et al., 2005; Thill et al., 2012). Similarly, imitation is also a major problem for children with autism, where the child has to imitate the response of the robot and in turn, the robot evaluates the imitated behaviour of the child (Feng et al., 2016; Scassellati, 2005).

2.6. EFFECT OF ROBOTIC PLATFORM

Any robotic interventions that aim to improve the engagement and communication skills of children (Maenner et al., 2014) and physical features (e.g. size, shape and looks of the embodiment) are of great importance in robotic therapeutic interventions (King & Bearman, 2009). These robotic features affect the behaviour of children with autism (CDC, 2022). Considering the findings, the clinical application of anthropomorphic and zoomorphic also categorised as humanoid and non-humanoid robots indicates promising development. In ASD, numerous types of non-humanoid, semi-humanoid and humanoid robots are available for this purpose. However, the main two categories are humanoid and non-humanoid robots (Ricks & Colton, 2010). Further under the category of humanoid robots, there are two types of robots: android and mechanical. Android robots look like humans and are repeatable and predictable in their tasks. Although they do have the capability of generalising tasks, children with autism are usually least interested towards these kinds of robots (Ricks & Colton, 2010). Another category of android robot is mascot robots that are cartoonish in their appearance while also maintaining their humanoid form. Mechanical robots are the ones that look like humans but are composed of mechanical parts that are dominant in their structure. Because of which children with ASD are more focussed towards the mechanical parts rather than interacting with the robot. Another category is of the non-humanoid mobile robots. These robots do not have a living appearance and therefore usually fail to imitate human–human interaction. Therefore, in therapeutic intervention for children with ASD, the focus is usually on the humanoid robots with which children are more involved during the interaction.

Design and form of the robot are considered as two important parameters when selecting it for therapeutic interventions. Different types of robotic embodiments are involved in therapeutic intervention for children with autism, where anthropomorphic robots (human look-alikes) are used for interventions based on social interaction and collaborative play (Tribune,

2022). The advantage of humanoid robots is that they have a capacity of generalisation such as imitation, emotion recognition, verbal correspondence, etc.

There is no unanimous consensus on the ideal appearance of a robot engaged in autism research, however, some fundamental recommendations for robot designs have been put forth by scientists. Researchers have studied the behaviour of children during interactions to note the significance of appearance. One such example is the research of Robins, Dautenhahn, Te Boekhorst, and Billard (2004) in which the doll-like robot Robota was given to the kids to engage with, both when it was dressed as a doll and when it was wearing basic white clothing and a sack over its head. It was concluded from this study that robots that communicate with autistic children should avoid a human's intricacy and minute details while maintaining their humanoid form. Famous anthropomorphic robots used for children with ASD are 'KASPAR' and 'NAO' (Landa, 2008; Shattuck, 2006). This technological intervention is preferred because of the robot's looks and predicably human-like nature, (Lintas & Persico, 2009) therefore, several features can increase the HRI (Dumont-Mathieu & Fein, 2005). Another well-known class of therapeutic robots are the ones that looks like animals, zoomorphic robots. One such robot for therapeutic interventions is 'Keepon' which is used for positive social interaction in therapies (Constantino et al., 2003). Other famous zoomorphic robots include Pleo, Charlie, Roball, Muu, and Aibo. A long-term study with Paro, a famous zoomorphic robot, reveals a good improvement in human interaction, demonstrating a significant role in therapy performance (Rutter, Bailey, et al., 2003). There are some other famous non-humanoid robots such as Robota Doll and Tito, etc. Whether anthropomorphic or zoomorphic robots, the predictable, safe, simple and reliable environment provided during robotic intervention makes the interaction different from humans.

Many of the researchers have also used non-humanoid robots for the interaction with ASD children. The simplicity of design allows the researchers to concentrate on building interesting and appealing interactions for children. One such robot is developed at the USC Interaction Lab called as Bandit Bubble Blowing Robot. The focus was not to make a human-like appearance but to develop an interactive task for children with autism (Feil-Seifer & Mataric, 2008b). Similarly, another robot named as Labo-1 that plays game of tag with children was developed by the researchers at University of Hertfordshire (Dautenhahn & Werry, 2004). Although the robots that take the appearance of animals, vehicles or toys do not elicit the same reactions as seen when interacting with humanoid robots, non-humanoid robots are easier to use and typically more affordable.

2.7. PROS AND CONS OF RATs

The use of interactive robots in therapy for children with ASD is a distinctive approach that has received significant attention in the research world. Robotic therapies have helped a lot in building the communication skills of children with ASD because a child is more inclined towards robots than humans and robots are more consistent and relatively immune to fatigue, unlike humans. Usually in these therapies, the improvement in impairment is noted using sensors, therefore, even the smallest improved behaviour can be noted compared with the ability of the naked eye. However, a lot of the work is evolving for integrating robots in clinical use for the improvement of skills and therefore a lot of improvement in the design of therapeutic intervention is needed. The design and effectiveness of the robotic platform are considered in detail, but the therapeutic protocol has received very little scrutiny (ASHA, 2022). The therapies usually have two to four persons in the intervention area including one controlling the robot. This arrangement is not considered feasible for clinical applications. In an ideal situation, the robot should be controlled by the therapist (whether within the intervention room or outside) by integrating technology with the software. A robot itself in the presence of the therapist should be studied as a co-presence during the treatment (Cardon, 2016). Mostly, the therapies are focussing on the improvement of behaviour. Very few therapies are based on the cognitive development of children with ASD targeting robot versus human interactions. One of the main problems with these therapies is that children with autism who might have the same score on the autism rating scale are very different from each other. Therefore, one therapy that can be useful for a particular child might not be generalisable. Therefore, introducing adaptive therapies that customise themselves according to the child's individual need will be beneficial. Very few such therapies exist and only for a few impairments. Moreover, triadic interaction should be promoted in these therapies to avoid the isolation of the child.

In Chapter 3, we consider the effects of various robotic therapies on families and society. This chapter will introduce and summarise the efficacy and impact of robotic intervention so far, as well as the sociopsychological and physiological implications of RAT for children with autism. This will go through the different aspects that influence the improvement of communication skills in children with ASD, as well as the factors that influence the child's adherence to, and acceptance of, robotic intervention. The chapter will present the impact of therapies so that future intervention techniques can be developed for improving communication skills (verbal and non-verbal), joint attention, imitation and behavioural aspects, including the impact of cultural differences in children's interactions with robots.

3

IMPLICATIONS OF ROBOT-ASSISTED THERAPIES ON CHILDREN WITH ASD

This chapter will discuss the role of robots that are operational within a human-inhabited setting. The latest and emerging circumstantial evidence indicates that the use of social robots has a unique impact on the improvement in social skills of children with ASD. This chapter will introduce and summarise the efficiency and impact of robotic intervention done so far including sociopsychological and physiological effects of RAT for children with autism. The critical analysis will be useful for all stakeholders associated with the field of RATs for children with ASD, such as psychologists, parents, students studying HRI and practitioners. It will compare various important factors that affect the improvement in communication skills of children with ASD including the factors for adherence and acceptability of robotic intervention by a child. It will also discuss the impact of robot therapeutic intervention on families of children with ASD. Moreover, it will present the impact on learning opportunities, and the effectiveness of social robots in teaching, evaluating the impact by assessing the attention, engagement, anxiety, and disruptive and repetitive behaviour of the child with autism.

The goal of this chapter is to present the impact of therapies so that they can help design future intervention techniques for improving communication skills (verbal and non-verbal), joint attention, imitation and behavioural aspects. The impact of cultural differences in children's interaction with robots, and how it could affect their behavioural learning using robots will also be discussed, along with the roles and functions of robots in human society and their implications from research in autism therapy.

3.1. ROLES OF ROBOTS IN RAATs

What are the expectations in terms of cognitive and behavioural competencies from a social robot that has to co-exist in human society? For this it is necessary to know the role of the robot in the community, may it be interaction with humans or task-based operation. Initially, robots were used for a limited task-based operation without interacting with humans. The concept of social robotics evolved over a period. Even in those task-based robotic operations humans were interacting with the robot as an operator or controlling personnel, just like a relationship with any other machine being operated by humans (Dautenhahn, 2003). A social robot, it is defined as a socially intelligent agent that shows characteristics of human intelligence.

In the context of the application area of autism, these robots develop an interaction based on the type of characteristics a particular autistic child lacks that can include qualitative impairment in social interaction, qualitative impairment in communication (verbal as well as non-verbal), restricted repetitive and stereotyped patterns of behaviour, interests and activities (Dautenhahn, 2003). There are different roles of robots in therapeutic interventions for children with ASD. Robots are usually considered as persuasive machines or therapeutic playmates such as in the Aurora project where one-to-one interaction of child–robot scenario was considered (Dautenhahn, 2001; Dautenhahn & Werry, 2000). In this role of the robot as a persuasive machine, it is defined as a therapeutic teaching device/tool used to teach basic social skills to children with autism. The second role that a robot can have in therapy is to be used as a tool to encourage and facilitate social behaviour among children. In this role, the robot is considered a social mediator that mediates the communication and interpersonal skills of children. However, designing a mediator robot requires careful study of how the children are interacting with different types of robots and how their capabilities and skills are being improved, what can be a particular desired interaction for any specific child that can help the children in any interaction scenario rather than only in the intervention room. Another role can be in terms of a social agent, acting as a surrogate for roles present in their environment and surroundings including parents, carers and other people in their social circle. If we use these social robots as social 'actors', this can help act out social stories, for observation, making them learn the social structure by acting (Dautenhahn, 2003). The robot as a social agent will be comparable to theatre-in-education (TIE) initiatives, where they perform educational stories so that audience can relate from a better perspective. In this case, when a robot will be acting as a social agent the task will be improvised based on the HRI rather than just like a theatre play where the actor is working with the already written script. This is how robots can add the element of interactivity rather than being akin to a normal puppet theatre show. Particularly in the case of autism, the child develops an attachment with the robot after a few interventions. Therefore, the robot becomes like a member of that group. It involves several challenging problems in terms of robot design, design of the 'play', and designing the interactive aspects of involving the child. However, the problem of a robot being a social actor is not simple. It involves several difficulties in terms of the design of the robot, designing the play itself keeping in view the child's requirement and involvement in interaction. Moreover, there is a certain limitation of each hardware that also needs to be kept in mind while designing the task for that social actor. The role of the robot is important as a social actor, which plays an important element in the child's development (Scassellati et al., 2012).

For this purpose, knowledge of interdisciplinary fields that includes robotics, psychology, cultural studies, social sciences and AI is required. These methods require diversified knowledge sources and skills that can be put together to form a successful application of any HRI.

3.1.1. Effect of Home-Based Robotic Therapies

Home-based robotic therapies are usually deployed, with autonomous robots having easier functional operation with simple mechanisms (Rakhymbayeva, Amirova, & Sandygulova, 2021). A therapeutic environment at home is the best-suited example for long-term studies (Baraka, Alves-Oliveira, & Ribeiro, 2020). In-home interventions are very common in autism therapies. Different interventions with both zoomorphic as well as anthropomorphic robots have been created. Pakkar, Clabaugh, Lee, Deng, and Matarićć (2019) designed an intervention for ASD children for over 1 month focussing on educational and social activities. The proposed system had a positive rating by both children as well as their parents. In another hierarchical human–robot learning (hHRL) study, a home-based therapy was proposed by Clabaugh et al. (2019) to improve the learning experience of children with ASD, where the proposed framework was regarded effective after 100 trials.

Research by Scassellati et al. looked at home-based therapy introducing games by the Jibo robot. The therapy focussed on multiple aspects including sequencing skills, perspective-taking, emotional understanding and many more (Scassellati et al., 2018). In all of the home-based robot therapies, children stayed engaged and showed improvement because of robotic therapies. However, for home-based interventions, family environment and occasional technical issues remain a problem. Moreover, the time for which a home-based therapy should be observed is also variable and no such generalised rule is yet followed.

3.2. EVALUATION STUDIES

Design, appearance and interaction protocols are some of the important factors in HRI, especially for autism. However, evaluation studies that show whether the developed protocol can achieve the intended goals or not are also important. Moreover, these evaluation studies should consider the optimal time for a certain therapy using robots. Currently, all the designed studies use their available robot without having any standards for making the design interaction protocol such as type of participants, experimental paradigm, affordability, number of interactions, size of sample size, hardware platform, structured or free-form interaction, and optimal time required for a certain therapy. Moreover, the standards of analysing data also vary and hence the conclusions. For example, the sample size is one of the important factors in these studies, where increasing the sample size ensures the validity of the data. Sample size is also dependent on the type of robot, as some robots allow free-form playgroups in which the researcher can observe several children at the same time, therefore increasing the sample set. Structured interaction trials and free-form interaction trials affect the results of an intervention. As the name reflects, a structured trial has an adult (a therapist, parent, or teacher) to conduct a study of the interaction between a child and the robot, whereas in free-form research there is no pre-defined task for child–robot interaction. Similarly, the difference in data analysis also changes the effect of an intervention. Two main categories of data analysis are quantitative and qualitative. Qualitative analysis is based on descriptive accounts, whereas quantitative analysis is usually analysed using statistical tools. The research shows that there are varieties of methods for addressing the same impairment using different platforms, sample sizes, and structured or free-form interactions without any standardisation.

Mostly the control architecture of therapies relies on behaviour-based design (Arkin, 1992). The advantage of this kind of system is that it responds effectively in time to social cues. The blending of different behaviours along with the external input from sensors can also be easily accommodated in such architecture. However, behaviour-based architecture for robotic therapies can be best implemented in long-term planning and social modes such as linguistic interaction as this model is not predictive and therefore cannot predict the child's response in upcoming interactions (Thill et al., 2012).

3.3. EFFECTS OF LONG- AND SHORT-TERM INTERACTIONS

These studies are also dependent on the number of interactions of an autistic child with the robot. As the child with autism is very sensitive to any new stimulus or change in the routine by the robotic intervention, we call this adaptability according to the child's need. Therefore, the amount of time the child has been exposed to a certain robotic interaction is an important factor. This time will affect the behaviour of the child for a certain intervention, depending on the specific platform. This is because the response of the child to the same stimulus will vary as the interaction of the robotic platform becomes familiar to him/her. Both interactions, long-term repeated interactions and short-term single interactions come with merits and weaknesses.

As far as short-term interactions are concerned, they are simpler, easier and less complex to perform logistically. Because there are typically fewer experimental trials, more participants can be recruited for that study, improving the validity of experiments. Moreover, the design of simpler experiments also confirms the usefulness of interaction and how the robot is treated by the child during an interaction. This further leads towards the useful design of interaction modelling as well as the design of the robot itself. In some studies, the novelty is also fostered through a familiarisation period during which participants and robots interact before the experiment (Feil-Seifer & Matarić, 2009).

However, if we consider the advantages of long-term/repeated interactions, it includes better tracking of HRI and data collection as the user has a certain given time to adjust to the robot (Dautenhahn et al., 2009; Kozima, Nakagawa, & Yasuda, 2007; Miyamoto, Lee, Fujii, & Okada, 2005; Robins, Dautenhahn, et al., 2004; Robins et al., 2005). Although interaction over time will be dependent on the child's mood and it will show how the robotic interaction can evolve with time (Scassellati et al., 2012). Studies with long-term interaction show that pro-social behaviour occurs after multiple interactions between the child and the robot. However, other dependent variables in a child's attitude including the effect of other interventions and maturity in a child's attitude with time shall also be considered.

3.4. EVOLVING CONCERNS

The socio-emotional bonding of children with ASD is different than a TD child. This engagement is considered a key factor for evaluating the quality of interaction. However, for all therapies, clinical or home-based, the goals of these interventions are to create therapies that are less intimidating for children with ASD, so that the response is better. However, the concept of engagement in research can be interpreted very differently. It can be defined in terms of attention, involvement, interest, absorption, rapport, empathy and posture that are used interchangeably and dynamically in the context of engagement (Salam, Celiktutan, Hupont, Gunes, & Chetouani, 2016). For this purpose, usually in research-based intervention triad interaction is noticed, this is because researchers think the engagement of the child in normal social scenarios should be the focus.

Another issue is the autonomy of the robotic intervention from a technical perspective. Accessing a child's response beyond WOZ should be considered (Scassellati et al., 2012). Though the fully autonomous model is unrealistic, a semi-autonomous model in which a robot user (e.g. therapist or researcher) might give instructions to a robot to achieve a certain set of goals and the robot, in turn, operate autonomously. Robot autonomy is an important focus of HRI in autism therapies. Experts suggest that these interventions shall be built around semi/fully autonomous robotic therapies with a more sophisticated robotic system (Anzalone et al., 2019; Melo et al., 2019; Rudovic, Lee, Mascarell-Maricic, Schuller, & Picard, 2017). Currently, almost all the robotic therapies are implementing the WOZ approach in which a human operator is controlling the robot but to the child it seems to be autonomous (Landauer, 1986; Wilson & Rosenberg, 1988). This might be a quick way for robotic therapy for immediate benefit without focussing on sophisticated intervention techniques (Thill et al., 2012). Few of the RAATs are using autonomous interaction but are still not being adaptive by fine-tuning the parameters of the algorithm based on child–robot interaction. Current algorithms do not focus on a child-centred approach for adapting the algorithms according to the child's behaviour, rather the proposed therapies are focussing on robotic technology (Wood, Zaraki, Robins, & Dautenhahn, 2019). Another main issue for researchers is the methodological constraints such as recruitment and retention plus experimental impediments including platform limitations (Rakhymbayeva et al., 2021). In the 'field' scenario, the evaluation of social skill improvement using robotic therapies requires better tools for data collection (Leite, Martinho, & Paiva, 2013). Moreover, over a period, interaction for improving a similar set of skills seems to be monotonous and repetitive, resulting in the reduction of a child's social engagement. Therefore, an optimal time for robotic interventions should be proposed. This might be compensated by focussing on building adaptive/autonomous robotic therapies based on user characteristics and personalisation as it will alter according to the child's requirement and need. Therefore, experimentation should be designed so to focus on an individualised research approach to meet a child's requirement according to his/her needs. Incorporating therapy recommendations by parents, child or therapists during the intervention can also be helpful for better design interventions.

Another important factor is data collection, which is usually done manually and charted or graphed over time. Even researchers have similar ways of manually collecting the data from intervention using biomarkers and analysing the video feeds. The aim of these technological interventions is that data for a child's improvement will be collected based on sensor recording rather than manual recording. This will ensure the reliability of data and will help parents and researchers to improve over time.

Furthermore, studies are highly dependent on the number of subjects recruited in an intervention. If a small number of subjects exist for an experiment, the intervention will not be considered (Pennisi et al., 2016). However, a higher number of subjects involved in any experiments will consequently lead to the acceptance of the hypothesis.

3.5. FUTURE DIRECTION

There are several broad methodological considerations for future studies that will aid in the interpretation of findings and the clinical relevance of these studies, especially the study that attempts to use robots for diagnostic objectives. To account for inherent variation in community diagnoses, these studies must align with the accepted diagnostic procedures. For this purpose, groups should be evaluated properly for their cognitive conditions to incorporate proper targeted therapeutic intervention.

A thorough empirical study that indicates the incremental authenticity of this approach over the available traditional methods should be conducted. This will also highlight the generalisation of robot-acquired skills versus those acquired through human interaction. Studies should also investigate whether having a robot in clinical setup ultimately improves interaction or could be replaced by other visually stimulated options such as videos, etc. One of the ways to approach this objective is to implement ABA therapies and integrate the robot into an empirically supported treatment for ASD (Liu, Conn, Sarkar, & Stone, 2008). Comparing the human–human interaction, pre- and post-intervention can also show the improvement done by therapeutic robotic interventions (Ali, et al., 2019). Every child with ASD has different therapeutic requirements, so instead of looking into what kind of robot should be used, the focus should be on how a child can gain the best out of these interventions. To achieve this, it is necessary to analyse the individual in groups based on their impairments so the approach can be tailored according to the individual's requirement.

Where the design of the robot has received much attention, the therapeutic requirement for this approach tends to lack formal guidelines and policies. In many of the interventions, the setup is neither practical nor economical for clinical applications. The number of people present in the intervention scenario are not constant. Similarly, for RAATs, the robot might be considered a peer to the therapist. The inclusion of robots along with the clinical intervention rules is necessary for the improved efficacy of robotic interventions. Moreover, how the robots can help towards generalisation of skills for an ASD child is an important factor to be explored (Diehl, Schmitt, Villano, & Crowell, 2012).

4

POLICY RECOMMENDATIONS, SUSTAINABLE DEVELOPMENT GOALS AND ETHICAL CONSIDERATIONS FOR SOCIETY OF AUTISM

This chapter will focus on suggesting the future direction in terms of policy recommendations and alignment with Sustainable Development Goals (SDGs), keeping in view the ethical considerations for RATs. The policies and future directions focus on an interdisciplinary research approach, which will be beneficial for all cross-disciplinary domains to develop robotic intervention systems in the future. Socially Assistive Robots (SARs) have the potential to increase client engagement, while at the same time making it possible for therapists to provide a more interactive session for the subject when it might not be possible to go to autism centres for their sessions. This chapter will focus on factors such as benefits to clients, therapists, scientists, and the public if behaviour analysts and robotic design engineers work together for further policies and SDGs on therapeutic intervention using robots. Such recommendations and policies are necessary for robust and effective assisted therapies, which include addressing the cost, quality and access to other considerations involved. These policies will also discuss the issues related to accessibility, affordability, and administrative burden, along with the ethical consideration for robotic interventions. It will suggest policies for robust robotic therapies that can increase engagement while considering the visual appeal and ease of accessibility. While suggesting future directions and policies, consideration will be given to certain aspects such as interaction, safety, autonomy, modularity, acceptability by both parents and child and adaptability. The goal of this chapter is to help scientists and policymakers to understand how digital technologies might help them achieve the SDGs and which ones will be most important in 2030. Moreover, it will summarise the policies and future directions for technological interventions using social robots that will be an affordable and effective option and can be incorporated to increase access, affordability, consistent services, and will reduce the administrative burden on therapists as well as parents. However, all of this shall be done under the umbrella of ethical consideration while dealing with children with autism.

4.1. INTRODUCTION

The rapidly advancing fields of AI, nanotechnology, and fields of communication and information are emerging into a new world for every individual, with lots of opportunities in both research and development (Pulsiri & Vatananan-Thesenvitz, 2018). The rise in population is causing an increase in the number of people with disabilities. Digital technology has been used for the improvement of the quality of life for disabled people and a more sustainable future through the United Nations' SDGs framework (Pulsiri et al., 2019). The digital technologies introduced for helping the disabled will contribute to the attainability of these SDGs. This chapter highlights the importance of mutual collaboration between scientists and policymakers on digital technology for better results towards targets. Planning of new policies, SDGs and business models is the focus of every growing nation (Schaller, Vatananan-Thesenvitz, & Stefania, 2018). UN Agenda 2030, which incorporates the 17 SDGs, addresses a better future for disabled people (U. N. G. Assembly, 2015). Moreover, research is now targeting the intervention following the UNICEF guidelines on AI for children (Lemaignan, Newbutt, Rice, Daly, & Charisi, 2021). For this purpose, research projects are used as a testbed to inculcate the significance and suitability of UNICEF guidelines on AI for Children. These targets support several UN goals for sustainable development keeping in view the well-being and emotional regulation of children with disabilities.

With respect to autism, children with ASD have more issues related to anxiety, depression, anger, etc. that ultimately have an impact on their education and personal life. A lot of research has been done on technology-based intervention for children with autism (Vahabzadeh et al., 2018; Williams & Gilbert, 2020), but none has focussed on including the users in the loop. Research has primarily begun to move towards an approach that includes autistic people in the design, development and evaluation of research about them rather than on autistic children themselves. Also, the ethical aspect during the intervention is considered according to the nature of autistic children (Schmidt, Newbutt, Schmidt, & Glaser, 2021), e.g. interventions shall be designed keeping in view how a non-verbal child can communicate easily (Lebenhagen, 2020) making the research meaningful (Parsons, Yuill, Good, & Brosnan, 2020; Zervogianni et al., 2020). The ground-breaking UNICEF report on AI and children, entitled 'Policy guidance on AI for children' layouts nine standards for designing AI systems aimed towards children (Dignum, Penagos, Pigmans, & Vosloo, 2020).

This chapter will now further elaborate on the ethical standards set by UNICEF and incorporate those in the policy recommendations along with the SDGs.

4.2. POLICY GUIDANCE BY UNICEF

The following nine standards are set by UNICEF for designing any AI system for children:

1. Focussing on the child's development and well-being while designing the system,
2. Ensuring inclusion of children,
3. Fair and non-discriminative behaviour for every child shall be ensured,
4. Protection of child's data and privacy,
5. Ensuring child's safety,
6. Transparency, accountability, and expansibility for every child,
7. Empowering government and business with the concept of AI along with children's rights,
8. Awareness of AI in children for the present and future,
9. Forming an enabling environment.

Even though, these recent advancements in AI extended the opportunities for children's well-being, they also accompanied additional concerns about increasing risks to children's rights. Considering this concern, UNICEF published these guidelines with several matching foci on child's individuality (Lemaignan et al., 2021), which provides a comprehensive framework with compact guidelines for designing any AI system for children. These guidelines oblige the designer to think about the end-user need, circumstances and environment in which the AI system will be deployed. The aim is to help develop better policymaking and research in the field of AI through considering the child's rights. However, emerging issues related to robotics are partially focussed on these guidelines, e.g. risks concerning the embodied nature of robotic artefacts for children. Some previous work on the ethics of child–robot interaction will be discussed later including the intersection of ethical considerations for robots and children with ASD.

As the research discussed in the previous chapters clearly states that there is an effect of robotic embodiment on a child's development and communication skills, therefore ethical consideration and possible risks associated with the embodiment should be regarded right from the beginning of designing the interaction. As these robots are dynamic objects and can move around in the physical environment of a child, safety, privacy and autonomy must be ensured. Organised and systematic assessments of ethical considerations in research for child–robot interaction still need to be gathered in a meaningful way. For now, the ethics are anticipatory in the sense that research must anticipate how these technologies will be applied in future and what will be the outcome (Brey, 2012; Johnson, 2007). This design challenge can, however, be addressed by involving parents, autism clinicians and educators right from the beginning of the design process (Alcorn, et al., 2019; Huijnen, Lexis, Jansens, & de Witte, 2017; Tolksdorf & Rohlfing, 2020). This will lead towards ensuring the second point in the guideline provided by UNICEF, i.e. 'ensure inclusion of and for children'. Moreover, considering the participation of autistic children during the design process also requires a link between pre-established broader ethical principles/guidelines and micro-ethics embodied within the application context (Spiel, Brulé, Frauenberger, Bailly, & Fitzpatrick, 2018). Until now only one researcher has implemented the UNICEF guidelines while designing an interaction of the robot with autistic children (Lemaignan et al., 2021). This research clearly explains how each of the nine principles of UNICEF has been implemented in their interaction. Principle 1, for example, the support of children's well-being and development is addressed by ensuring that the robot provides social support only to people who ask for it and these social needs were identified from in-school focus groups and their teachers. Another example is Principle 5 'ensuring safety during the interaction'. This was done by training the on-site researcher and school staff to recognise distress during the intervention. In this way, UNICEF guidelines are closely aligned with a user-centred approach based on a strong ethical framing. To support the implementation of guidelines and address the complexities, UNICEF has encouraged governments and the business sector to test these policy guidelines in various fields.

4.3. RESPONSIBLE AI IS ETHICAL

Efforts towards responsible, ethical, and trustworthy AI builds confidence among the users and is a subject of great interest. By taking this approach, proponents hope that governments and businesses will indulge more in the potential of AI models due to safer, ethical and more transparent approaches. Responsible AI entails ensuring that designed AI systems are ethical, legal, beneficial and robust. Moreover, these features can be verified, and those who deploy or use these systems are held accountable (Dignum, 2019). Each person involved in the AI development ecosystem must be aware of the critical concerns that must be addressed to contribute to responsible AI. This includes people who make the AI policies, people who design the AI algorithms, software programmers who build the system, individuals tagging data and finally those who are using the AI system for interaction. For a productive AI system, everyone in the chain should be informed about how, why and for what specific purpose the system is designed for.

Talking particularly about children with autism and robot-led therapies, researchers have presented an ethical analysis for the robot led therapies (Science Digital, 2022). This research analyses the ethics of robot deployments focussing on issues such as autonomy, community, transparency, identity, value, and empathy for robot-led therapeutic interventions.

4.3.1. AI and Child's Rights: Risk Versus Opportunities

On many forums of AI and child rights, youth are demanding that, along with privacy, their wellbeing is protected, and users are given the latest and authentic information that will help them as a child. For this idea, a chatbot was preferred where parents can guide them with their life decisions. In the case of the AI system, the questions that need to be addressed are: How it is designed? For what purpose it is used? and Can it undermine or uphold the child's rights? AI policies should work centrally around these concepts to protect child's rights. For the rights of children: protection, provision and involvement are the lenses that might be used to look at the situation. This should cover all the aspects related to a child's protection against discrimination, abuse, exploitation, privacy, etc. One of the main concerns of these therapies is that they focus on the robot a lot rather than the human himself. In terms of robot autonomy, this may be addressed by, rather than the robot telling the child to do a certain task, designing interactions so the child tells the robot (U. N. G. Assembly,

2015). This will ultimately give the child a better opportunity for autonomy and making decisions by managing the social complexity of the environment, keeping in view the ethical consideration to be practiced while doing robot led therapies. Technological ethics cannot be separated from social ethics, as the use of technology is derived from the purpose in society itself, and therefore cannot be isolated from each other. However, to improve the effect of technological interventions, the focus of these tech therapies should be shifted from robots to subjects. The active ethics led therapies focus on six main ethical areas: Autonomy, Community, Transparency, Identity, Value and Empathy (U. N. G. Assembly, 2015). The aim of these ethical concerns is mainly related to the fact that focusses on humans rather than robots. For example, in the case of autonomy, the interaction shall be initiated by the child rather than the robot, where a child should not feel that the robot is leading his/her behaviour.

To summarise the ethical concerns that should be implemented in future interventions, should be human centred in approach. Understanding what the child thinks and how he/she feels will enable the child to focus on communication rather than coping with emotional overload because of the presence of the robot. We must get inside the mind of the autistic child and thereby set ethical boundaries and pursue ethical design based on our understanding of the autistic child.

4.4. DIGITAL TECHNOLOGIES AND SDGs FOR CHILDREN WITH DISABILITIES

Digital technology is increasingly being used to facilitate disabled people in Activities of Daily Life (ADL). The United Nations' SDGs framework focusses on the development of a brighter and more sustainable future using digital technologies. For this purpose, it is important to develop a connection between digital technologies and SDGs that will help to evaluate the potential of digital technologies and maximise their application for people with disabilities. This will also help researchers as well as policymakers to know how these technologies can address SDGs.

Where digital technologies can be used to solve multiple problems, there could be significant impact on stakeholders that should be assessed at the national level before the necessary investments in digital technology programs for the disabled are made (Pulsiri et al., 2019; Schaller et al., 2018). The use of these digital technologies will lead to human–machine interaction in near future which promise to facilitate humans in their daily activities and help with most physical limitations encountered by the disabled person (WHO, 2007).

According to the definition of the WHO, the phrase 'disabilities' refers to impairments, activity constraints and participation restrictions (Kaplan, 1999). In this approach, disability does not refer to the health problems and physical limitations only but also encompasses the human mind along with other features of society (Lederer, Loisel, Rivard, & Champagne, 2014). At present, there are seven main types of disabilities, i.e. visual disability, hearing, or communication disability, physical or locomotion disability, mental or behavioural disability, intellectual disability, learning disability and autism (U. N. G. Assembly, 2015). To include them in society and make them independent in their daily life activities, it is necessary to include them in the SDG framework. To achieve the aim of including everyone, the 2030 Agenda for Sustainable Development, with its 17 SDGs, has been designed as a powerful framework for countries and the international community to follow on their way to universal peace and better freedom (McBride, 2020).

The combination of robots and AI opens a world of solutions and opportunities which were impossible to achieve in the recent past. Solution that can analyse, react and adapt to the environment can help in achieving the United Nations' SDGs.

Another major concern for individuals with ASD is unemployment or underemployment. National data indicates that the concern of these individuals is genuine (Cardon, 2016). Individuals with autism deserve to have better opportunities where they can contribute in suitable settings. Moreover, studies have confirmed that individuals with ASD usually drop out of college similar reasons as unpaid jobs. The obstacles for jobs include sensory challenges, office misperceptions, inability to work in group, understanding and dealing with office politics, considered different by their co-workers, stress because of unpredictability, etc. It can also have significant economic implications on parental employments and also on earning in terms of parental labour force participation, hours of work and annual earnings (Cidav, Marcus, & Mandell, 2012). Therefore, it is necessary to design universal policies in the workplace as well as educational institutions that cater for the requirements and health benefits of individuals with ASD.

4.5. CONCLUSION

In the Industry 4.0 era, digitalisation has revolutionised our industries and social lives. Digital technology has intervened in learning as well to better provide children with opportunities and facilitating them to learn, grow and realise their potential. The support through digitalisation is inclusive of both

TD children and children with disabilities. It provides access to upgraded and more efficient intervention to connect children with their friends, better civic engagement, social inclusion, and other opportunities, potentially breaking the stereotypes of disability. The 2030 Agenda for Sustainable Development, with its 17 SDGs, has been designed as a powerful framework for countries and the international community to follow on their way to universal peace and greater freedom for everyone (Lord et al., 1997). As a result, ATs will be an essential tool to increase independence and participation in education, employment and access to the community for people with disabilities (Schopler et al., 1988). Assistive and digital technology are not limited to a certain type of product or intervention but include all products, equipment and systems that encompass both high-end and low-end devices, applications and technologies. WHO highlights that only 10% of people in need of AT have access to it. A major concern for policymakers, therefore, should be access to these ATs for everyone who needs it. Although the provision of ATs varies from country to country, the global focus should be the intent to facilitate the disabled community by fulfilling the potential of technological interventions.

Where the design of robot has received considerable attention, the focus of therapies should be around the therapeutic protocol of the RATs. Moreover, future research should not only focus on what kind of robot and how it should be used but rather it should move towards 'who' requires the robot based therapeutic interventions. It is important to establish which ASD impairments respond best towards these technological interventions. Building the research around whether characteristics like the intensity of social impairment, the prominence of stereotyped and repeated behaviours, sensory difficulties, or other significant aspects influence the effectiveness of therapy or not is also important. This will eventually lead towards greater applicability and its adaptability to therapy for individuals with ASD.

With the advancement in the technology and improved understanding of the brain dynamics of an ASD child, there is a chance for improved research to address the communication problems for any impairment of an ASD child. Data from early intervention results should be paired with innovative technologies in the form of software applications or other devices such as Brain–Computer Interface (BCI) (Ali, et al., 2019) to better analyse the improvement and access data over the time. Professional collaboration is essential for achieving the best results by offering their key expertise from the perspective of contributing unique knowledge in their specific domain area.

It is hard to foresee how technological advancements over the next 20 years may transform and affect the lives of people with ASD, but the possibilities seem genuinely endless if future technology develops even remotely as quickly and uniquely as it has in the previous 20 years.

This book tries to explain different kind of RATs focussing on various impairments along with their effectiveness. Moreover, the development of future policies that will be needed to account for shifting boundaries between humans and machines as they are re-formed through new technologies and practices in developing RATs. However, we also emphasise that with all the technological advancements, one cannot neglect the importance of human nature. In this regard, a few unanswered issues remain, for example, the implications of claims that most human medical experts will eventually be replaced by robots, especially in the context of therapies for children with ASD. Moreover, the generalised/standardised use of therapies needs further research as each child with ASD has different challenges and thus each child should be given different therapies. Moreover, the cost of a humanoid robot is still a big question mark when parents and therapy centres think of moving towards robotic interventions, although robots are increasingly being promoted as viable therapy products. However, if the focus is for them to replace humans and intimate relationships, then proper ethical considerations must be kept in regard while promoting robot technology. Therefore, a lot of effort is still required for enabling human–machine interaction to replace human–human interaction, as 'using a robot' and 'being with a robot' are entirely different concepts linked with ontological differences between humans and machines.

REFERENCES

Abrahams, B. S., & Geschwind, D. H. (2008). Advances in autism genetics: On the threshold of a new neurobiology. *Nature Reviews Genetics*, *9*(5), 341–355.

Adams, A., & Robinson, P. (2011). An android head for social-emotional intervention for children with autism spectrum conditions. In *International conference on affective computing and intelligent interaction* (pp. 183–190).

Alcorn, A. M., Ainger, E., Charisi, V., Mantinioti, S., Petrović, S., Schadenberg, B. R., Tavassoli, T., & Pellicano, E. (2019). Educators' views on using humanoid robots with autistic learners in special education settings in England. *Frontiers in Robotics and AI*, 6, 107.

Alemi, M., Meghdari, A., Basiri, N. M., & Taheri, A. (2015). The effect of applying humanoid robots as teacher assistants to help Iranian autistic pupils learn English as a foreign language. In *International conference on social robotics* (pp. 1–10).

Ali, S., Mehmood, F., Dancey, D., Ayaz, Y., Khan, M. J., Naseer, N., de Cassia Amadeu, R., Sadia, H., & Nawaz, R. (2019). An adaptive multi-robot therapy for improving joint attention and imitation of ASD Children. *IEEE Access*.

Ali, S., Mehmood, F., Ayaz, Y., Khan, M. J., Sadia, H., & Nawaz, R. (2020). Comparing the effectiveness of different reinforcement stimuli in a robotic therapy for children with ASD. *IEEE Access*, *8*, 13128–13137. doi: 10.1109/ACCESS.2020.2965204

Ali, S., Mehmood, F., Ayaz, Y., Sajid, M., Sadia, H., & Nawaz, R. (2022, June). An experimental trial: Multi-robot therapy for categorization of autism level using hidden Markov Model. *Journal of Educational Computing Research*, *60*(3), 722–741. doi: 10.1177/07356331211040405

American Psychiatric Association and Others. (1980). *Diagnostic and statistical manual of mental disorders* (Vol. 3). Washington, DC: American Psychiatric Association.

American Psychiatric Association and Others. (2013). Diagnostic and statistical manual of mental disorders. *BMC Medicine*, *17*, 133–137.

Anzalone, S. M., Xavier, J., Boucenna, S., Billeci, L., Narzisi, A., Muratori, F., ... Chetouani, M. (2019). Quantifying patterns of joint attention during human–robot interactions: An application for autism spectrum disorder assessment. *Pattern Recognition Letters*, *118*, 42–50.

Arkin, R. C. (1992). Homeostatic control for a mobile robot: Dynamic replanning in hazardous environments. *Journal of Robotic Systems*, *9*(2), 197–214.

ASHA. (2022). American Speech-Language-Hearing Association | ASHA. Retrieved from https://www.asha.org/. Accessed on July 06, 2022.

Bai, S., Repetti, R. L., & Sperling, J. B. (2016). Children's expressions of positive emotion are sustained by smiling, touching, and playing with parents and siblings: A naturalistic observational study of family life. *Developmental Psychology*, *52*(1), 88.

Baraka, K., Alves-Oliveira, P., & Ribeiro, T. (2020). An extended framework for characterizing social robots, 21–64. doi: 10.1007/978-3-030-42307-0_2

Bauminger, N. (2002). The facilitation of social-emotional understanding and social interaction in high-functioning children with autism: Intervention outcomes. *Journal of Autism and Developmental Disorders*, *32*(4), 283–298.

Bharatharaj, J., Huang, L., Al-Jumaily, A., Elara, M. R., & Krägeloh, C. (2017). Investigating the effects of robot-assisted therapy among children with autism spectrum disorder using bio-markers. *IOP Conference Series: Materials Science and Engineering*, *234*(1), 1.

Bleuler, E. (1912). The theory of schizophrenic negativism. *Journal of Nervous and Mental Disease Publishing Company*, no. 11.

Botha, M., & Frost, D. M. (2020). Extending the minority stress model to understand mental health problems experienced by the autistic population. *Society and Mental Health*, *10*(1), 20–34.

Breazeal, C. (2009). Role of expressive behaviour for robots that learn from people. *Philosophical Transactions of the Royal Society B*, *364*(1535), 3527–3538.

Brey, P. A. E. (2012). Anticipatory ethics for emerging technologies. *Nanoethics*, *6*(1), 1–13.

Buffington, D. M., Krantz, P. J., McClannahan, L. E., & Poulson, C. L. (1998). Procedures for teaching appropriate gestural communication skills to children with autism. *Journal of Autism and Developmental Disorders, 28*(6), 535–545.

Buxbaum, J. D. (2009). Multiple rare variants in the etiology of autism spectrum disorders. *Dialogues in Clinical Neuroscience, 11*(1), 35.

Cardon, T. A. (Ed.). (2016). *Technology and the treatment of children with autism spectrum disorder*. doi: 10.1007/978-3-319-20872-5

Caronna, E. B., Milunsky, J. M., & Tager-Flusberg, H. (2008). Autism spectrum disorders: Clinical and research frontiers. *Archives of Disease in Childhood, 93*(6), 518–523.

Carter, C., Meckes, L., Pritchard, L., Swensen, S., Wittman, P. P., & Velde, B. (2004). The friendship club: An after-school program for children with Asperger syndrome. *Family & Community Health, 27*(2), 143–150.

Cascio, C. J., Gu, C., Schauder, K. B., Key, A. P., & Yoder, P. (2015). Somatosensory event-related potentials and association with tactile behavioral responsiveness patterns in children with ASD. *Brain Topography, 28*(6), 895–903.

Cascio, C. J., Lorenzi, J., & Baranek, G. T. (2016). Self-reported pleasantness ratings and examiner-coded defensiveness in response to touch in children with ASD: Effects of stimulus material and bodily location. *Journal of Autism and Developmental Disorders, 46*(5), 1528–1537.

Centers for Disease Control and Prevention (CDC). (2022). Key Findings: CDC Releases First Estimates of the Number of Adults Living with Autism Spectrum Disorder in the United States | Autism | NCBDDD | CDC. Retrieved from https://www.cdc.gov/ncbddd/autism/features/adults-living-with-autism-spectrum-disorder.html. Accessed on February 22, 2022.

Chernyak, N., & Gary, H. E. (2016). Children's cognitive and behavioral reactions to an autonomous versus controlled social robot dog. *Early Education and Development, 27*(8), 1175–1189.

Chiang, I.-T., Lee, Y., Frey, G., & McCormick, B. (2004). Testing the situationally modified social rank theory on friendship quality in male youth with high-functioning autism spectrum disorder. *Therapeutic Recreation Journal, 38*(3), 261.

Chlebowski, C., Green, J. A., Barton, M. L., & Fein, D. (2010). Using the childhood autism rating scale to diagnose autism spectrum disorders. *Journal of Autism and Developmental Disorders*, *40*(7), 787–799.

Cidav, Z., Marcus, S. C., & Mandell, D. S. (2012). Implications of childhood autism for parental employment and earnings. *Pediatrics*, *129*(4), 617. doi: 10.1542/PEDS.2011-2700

Clabaugh, C., Mahajan, K., Jain, S., Pakkar, R., Becerra, D., Shi, Z., … Matarić, M. (2019). Long-term personalization of an in-home socially assistive robot for children with autism spectrum disorders. *Frontiers in Robotics and AI*, *6*, 110.

Cohen, H., Amerine-Dickens, M., & Smith, T. (2006). Early intensive behavioral treatment: Replication of the UCLA model in a community setting. *Journal of Developmental and Behavioral Pediatrics*, *27*(2), S145–S155.

Constantino, J. N., Davis, S. A., Todd, R. D., Schindler, M. K., Gross, M. M., Brophy, S. L., … Reich, W. (2003). Validation of a brief quantitative measure of autistic traits: Comparison of the social responsiveness scale with the autism diagnostic interview-revised. *Journal of Autism and Developmental Disorders*, *33*(4), 427–433.

Dautenhahn, K. (2001). The AURORA project: Using mobile robots in autism therapy. *Learning Technologies*, *3*(1).

Dautenhahn, K. (2003). Roles and functions of robots in human society: Implications from research in autism therapy. *Robotica*, *21*(4), 443–452.

Dautenhahn, K., Nehaniv, C. L., Walters, M. L., Robins, B., Kose-Bagci, H., Assif Mirza, N., & Blow, M. (2009). KASPAR – A minimally expressive humanoid robot for human–robot interaction research. *Applied Bionics and Biomechanics*, 6(3–4), 369–397.

Dautenhahn, K., & Werry, I. (2000). Issues of robot-human interaction dynamics in the rehabilitation of children with autism. *Proc. From Animals to Animats* 6, 6(519–528), 25.

Dautenhahn, K., & Werry, I. (2004, January). Towards interactive robots in autism therapy: Background, motivation and challenges. *Pragmatics & Cognition*, *12*(1), 1–35. doi: 10.1075/PC.12.1.03DAU

Dawson, G., Rogers, S., Munson, J., Smith, M., Winter, J., Greenson, J., … Varley, J. (2010, January). Randomized, controlled trial of an intervention for toddlers with autism: The Early Start Denver Model. *Pediatrics*, *125*(1). doi: 10.1542/PEDS.2009-0958

Diehl, J. J., Schmitt, L. M., Villano, M., & Crowell, C. R. (2012). The clinical use of robots for individuals with autism spectrum disorders: A critical review. *Research in Autism Spectrum Disorders*, *6*(1), 249–262.

Dignum, V. (2019). *Responsible artificial intelligence: How to develop and use AI in a responsible way*. Springer Nature. Retrieved from https://link.springer.com/book/10.1007/978-3-030-30371-6#about-this-book

Dignum, V., Penagos, M., Pigmans, K., & Vosloo, S. (2020) *Policy guidance on AI for children*. Technical Report, UNICEF. Retrieved from https://www.unicef. org/globalinsight~...,

Dumont-Mathieu, T., & Fein, D. (2005). Screening for autism in young children: The Modified Checklist for Autism in Toddlers (M-CHAT) and other measures. *Mental Retardation and Developmental Disabilities Research*, *11*(3), 253–262.

Eikeseth, S. (2009). Outcome of comprehensive psycho-educational interventions for young children with autism. *Research in Developmental Disabilities*, *30*(1), 158–178.

Esteban, P. G., Baxter, P., Belpaeme, T., Billing, E., Cai, H., Cao, H.-L., ... Ziemke, T. (2017). How to build a supervised autonomous system for robot-enhanced therapy for children with autism spectrum disorder. *Paladyn. Journal of Behavioral Robotics*, *8*(1), 18–38.

EurekAlert. (2022). Socially assistive robot helps children with | EurekAlert! Retrieved from https://www.eurekalert.org/news-releases/610176. Accessed on February 23, 2022.

Feil-Seifer, D., & Mataric, M. J. (2008a). B [3] IA: A control architecture for autonomous robot-assisted behavior intervention for children with Autism Spectrum Disorders. In *RO-MAN 2008-The 17th IEEE international symposium on robot and human interactive communication* (pp. 328–333).

Feil-Seifer, D., & Mataric, M. (2008b). Robot-assisted therapy for children with Autism Spectrum Disorders. In *IDC '08: Proceedings of the 7th international conference on Interaction design and children* (pp. 49–52). doi: 10.1145/1463689.1463716

Feil-Seifer, D., & Matarić, M. J. (2009). Toward socially assistive robotics for augmenting interventions for children with autism spectrum disorders. In *Experimental robotics* (pp. 201–210).

Feng, Y., Jia, Q., Chen, G., & Li, C. (2016). Control architecture design for intelligent robot assisted intervention for children with autism. In *2016*

IEEE 11th conference on industrial electronics and applications (ICIEA) (pp. 1345–1349).

Fitzgerald, E., Yap, H. K., Ashton, C., Moore, D. W., Furlonger, B., Anderson, A., ... English, D. L. (2018, April). Comparing the effectiveness of virtual reality and video modelling as an intervention strategy for individuals with Autism Spectrum Disorder: Brief report. *Developmental Neurorehabilitation*, *21*(3), 197–201. doi: 10.1080/17518423.2018.1432713

Fombonne, E. (2009). Epidemiology of pervasive developmental disorders. *Pediatric Research*, *65*(6), 591–598.

Freitag, C. M. (2007). The genetics of autistic disorders and its clinical relevance: A review of the literature. *Molecular Psychiatry*, *12*(1), 2–22.

Frost, L., & Bondy, A. (2002). *The picture exchange communication system (PECS) Training Manual* (2nd ed.). Newark, DE. Pyramid Products, Inc. - Pyramid Educational Consultants Pyramid Educational Consultants. Retrieved from https://pecs.com/frost-l-bondy-a-2002-the-picture-exchange-communication-system-pecs-training-manual-2nd-edition-newark-de-pyramid-products-inc/. Accessed on July 06, 2022.

Geschwind, D. H. (2009). Advances in autism. *Annual Review of Medicine*, *60*, 367–380.

Happé, F. (1999). Understanding assets and deficits in autism: Why success is more interesting than failure. *The Psychologist*, *12*(11), 540–546.

Happé, F., & Ronald, A. (2008). The 'fractionable autism triad': A review of evidence from behavioural, genetic, cognitive and neural research. *Neuropsychology Review*, *18*(4), 287–304.

Happé, F., Ronald, A., & Plomin, R. (2006). Time to give up on a single explanation for autism. *Nature Neuroscience*, *9*(10), 1218–1220.

Hendricks, D. R., & Wehman, P. (2009). Transition from school to adulthood for youth with autism spectrum disorders: Review and recommendations. *Focus on Autism and Other Developmental Disabilities*, *24*(2), 77–88.

Howlin, P., Magiati, I., & Charman, T. (2009). Systematic review of early intensive behavioral interventions for children with autism. *American Journal on Intellectual and Developmental Disabilities*, *114*(1), 23–41.

Huijnen, C. A. G. J., Lexis, M. A. S., Jansens, R., & de Witte, L. P. (2017). How to implement robots in interventions for children with autism? A co-creation study involving people with autism, parents and professionals. *Journal of Autism and Developmental Disorders*, *47*(10), 3079–3096.

Israelyan, N., & Margolis, K. G. (2019). Reprint of: Serotonin as a link between the gut-brain-microbiome axis in autism spectrum disorders. *Pharmacological Research*, *140*, 115–120.

Ji, N. Y., & Findling, R. L. (2015). An update on pharmacotherapy for autism spectrum disorder in children and adolescents. *Current Opinion in Psychiatry*, *28*(2), 91–101.

Johnson, D. G. (2007). Ethics and technology 'in the making': An essay on the challenge of nanoethics. *Nanoethics*, *1*(1), 21–30.

Kanner, L. (1943). Autistic disturbances of affective contact. *Nervous Child*, *2*(3), 217–250.

Kaplan, D. (1999). The definition of disability: Perspective of the disability community. *Journal of Health Care Law and Policy*, *3*, 352.

Kasari, C., Freeman, S., & Paparella, T. (2006). Joint attention and symbolic play in young children with autism: A randomized controlled intervention study. *Journal of Child Psychology and Psychiatry*, *47*(6), 611–620.

Kim, E. S., Berkovits, L. D., Bernier, E. P., Leyzberg, D., Shic, F., Paul, R., & Scassellati, B. (2013). Social robots as embedded reinforcers of social behavior in children with autism. *Journal of Autism and Developmental Disorders*, *43*(5), 1038–1049.

King, M., & Bearman, P. (2009). Diagnostic change and the increased prevalence of autism. *International Journal of Epidemiology*, *38*(5), 1224–1234.

Kopp, S., & Gillberg, C. (2011). The Autism Spectrum Screening Questionnaire (ASSQ)-Revised Extended Version (ASSQ-REV): An instrument for better capturing the autism phenotype in girls? A preliminary study involving 191 clinical cases and community controls. *Research in Developmental Disabilities*, *32*(6), 2875–2888.

Kozima, H., Nakagawa, C., & Yasuda, Y. (2005). Interactive robots for communication-care: A case-study in autism therapy. In *ROMAN 2005. IEEE International Workshop on Robot and Human Interactive Communication* (pp. 341–346).

Kozima, H., Nakagawa, C., & Yasuda, Y. (2007). Children–robot interaction: A pilot study in autism therapy. *Progress in Brain Research*, *164*, 385–400.

Lahiri, U. (2020). *A computational view of autism*. Springer. Retrieved from https://link.springer.com/book/10.1007/978-3-030-40237-2#about-this-book

Lam, J., Sutton, P., Kalkbrenner, A., Windham, G., Halladay, A., Koustas, E., ... Woodruff, T. (2016). A systematic review and meta-analysis of multiple airborne pollutants and autism spectrum disorder. *PLoS One*, *11*(9), e0161851.

Landa, R. J. (2008). Diagnosis of autism spectrum disorders in the first 3 years of life. *Nature Reviews Neurology*, *4*(3), 138–147.

Landa, R. J., & Kalb, L. G. (2012). Long-term outcomes of toddlers with autism spectrum disorders exposed to short-term intervention. *Pediatrics*, *130*(Supplement 2), S186–S190.

Landauer, T. K. (1986). Psychology as a mother of invention. *ACM SIGCHI Bulletin*, *18*(4), 333–335.

Lebenhagen, C. (2020). Including speaking and nonspeaking autistic voice in research. *Autism in Adulthood*, 2(2), 128–131.

Lederer, V., Loisel, P., Rivard, M., & Champagne, F. (2014). Exploring the diversity of conceptualizations of work (dis) ability: A scoping review of published definitions. *Journal of Occupational Rehabilitation*, *24*(2), 242–267.

Leite, I., Martinho, C., & Paiva, A. (2013). Social robots for long-term interaction: A survey. *International Journal of Social Robotics*, *5*(2), 291–308.

Lemaignan, S., Newbutt, N., Rice, L., Daly, J., & Charisi, V. (2021). UNICEF Guidance on AI for Children: Application to the Design of a Social Robot For and With Autistic Children. *arXiv Prepr. arXiv2108.12166*.

Levy, S. E., Mandell, D. S., & Schultz, R. T. (2009). Autism. *The Lancet*, *374*(9701), 1627–1638.

Lintas, C., & Persico, A. M. (2009). Autistic phenotypes and genetic testing: State-of-the-art for the clinical geneticist. *Journal of Medical Genetics*, *46*(1), 1–8.

Liu, C., Conn, K., Sarkar, N., & Stone, W. (2008). Online affect detection and robot behavior adaptation for intervention of children with autism. *IEEE Transactions on Robotics*, *24*(4), 883–896.

London, E. (2007). The role of the neurobiologist in redefining the diagnosis of autism. *Brain Pathology*, *17*(4), 408–411.

Lord, C., Pickles, A., McLennan, J., Rutter, M., Bregman, J., Folstein, S., ... Minshew, N. (1997). Diagnosing autism: Analyses of data from the Autism Diagnostic Interview. *Journal of Autism and Developmental Disorders*, *27*(5), 501–517.

Lotter, V. (1967). Epidemiology of autistic conditions in young children. *Social Psychiatry*, *1*(4), 163–173.

Lovaas, O. I. (1987). Behavioral treatment and normal educational and intellectual functioning in young autistic children. *Journal of Consulting and Clinical Psychology*, *55*(1), 3.

Lyall, K., Schmidt, R. J., & Hertz-Picciotto, I. (2014). Maternal lifestyle and environmental risk factors for autism spectrum disorders. *International Journal of Epidemiology*, *43*(2), 443–464.

Mace, F. C. (1994). The significance and future of functional analysis methodologies. *Journal of Applied Behavior Analysis*, *27*(2), 385–392.

Maenner, M. J., Rice, C. E., Arneson, C. L., Cunniff, C., Schieve, L. A., Carpenter, L. A., ... Durkin, M. S. (2014). Potential impact of DSM-5 criteria on autism spectrum disorder prevalence estimates. *JAMA Psychiatry*, *71*(3), 292–300.

Maenner, M. J., Shaw, K. A., Baio, J., Washington, A., Patrick, M., DiRienzo, M., ... Dietz, P. M. (2020). Prevalence of autism spectrum disorder among children aged 8 years – Autism and developmental disabilities monitoring network, 11 sites, United States, 2016. *MMWR Surveillance Summaries*, *69*(4), 1.

Mammen, M. A., Moore, G. A., Scaramella, L. V., Reiss, D., Ganiban, J. M., Shaw, D. S., ... Neiderhiser, J. M. (2015). Infant avoidance during a tactile task predicts autism spectrum behaviors in toddlerhood. *Infant Mental Health Journal*, *36*(6), 575–587.

Marino, F., Chilà, P., Sfrazzetto, S. T., Carrozza, C., Crimi, I., & Failla, C. (2020). Outcomes of a robot-assisted social-emotional understanding intervention for young children with autism spectrum disorders. *Journal of Autism and Developmental Disorders*, *50*(6), 1973–1987.

McBride, N. (2020). Robot enhanced therapy for autistic children: An ethical analysis. *IEEE Technology and Society Magazine*, *39*(1), 51–60.

Mehmood, F., Ayaz, Y., Ali, S., De Cassia Amadeu, R., & Sadia, H. (2019). Dominance in visual space of ASD children using multi-robot joint attention integrated distributed imitation system. *IEEE Access*, 7, 168815–168827. doi: 10.1109/ACCESS.2019.2951366

Melo, F. S., Sardinha, A., Belo, D., Couto, M., Faria, M., Farias, A., ... Kinarullathil, M. (2019). Project INSIDE: Towards autonomous semi-unstructured human–robot social interaction in autism therapy. *Artificial Intelligence in Medicine*, *96*, 198–216.

Mesa-Gresa, P., Gil-Gómez, H., Lozano-Quilis, J. A., & Gil-Gómez, J. A. (2018, August). Effectiveness of virtual reality for children and adolescents with autism spectrum disorder: An evidence-based systematic review. *Sensors (Basel)*, *18*(8). doi: 10.3390/S18082486

MIT Technology Review. (2022). Robots that teach autistic kids social skills could help them develop | MIT Technology Review. Retrieved from https://www.technologyreview.com/2020/02/26/916719/ai-robots-teach-autistic-kids-social-skills-development/. Accessed on February 23, 2022.

Miyamoto, E., Lee, M., Fujii, H., & Okada, M. (2005). *How can robots facilitate social interaction of children with autism?: Possible implications for educational environments.*

Moore, S. T. (2002). *Asperger syndrome and the elementary school experience: Practical solutions for academic & social difficulties.* Shawnee, KS: AAPC Publishing.

Myers, S. M., Johnson, C. P., & American Academy of Pediatrics Council on Children With Disabilities. (2007). Management of children with autism spectrum disorders. *Pediatrics*, *120*(5), 1162–1182.

Nakabayashi, M., & Matsumoto, M. (2003). *Psychological tests and Asperger syndrome: The association with continuing facilitative assistance. Japanese Journal of Child and Adolescent Psychiatry*, *44*(5), 425–439.

Newschaffer, C. J., Croen, L. A., Daniels, J., Giarelli, E., Grether J. K., Levy, S. E., ... Windham, G. C. (2007). The epidemiology of autism spectrum disorders. *Annual Review of Public Health*, *28*, 235–258.

Ospina, M. B., Seida, J. K., Clark, B., Karkhaneh, M., Hartling, L., Tjosvold, L., ... Smith, V. (2008). Behavioural and developmental interventions for autism spectrum disorder: A clinical systematic review. *PLoS One*, *3*(11), e3755.

Pakkar, R., Clabaugh, C., Lee, R., Deng, E., & Mataricć, M. J. (2019). Designing a socially assistive robot for long-term in-home use for children with autism spectrum disorders. In *2019 28th IEEE International Conference on Robot and Human Interactive Communication (RO-MAN)* (pp. 1–7).

Parents. (2022). A Timeline of the History of Autism Spectrum Disorder. Retrieved from https://www.parents.com/health/autism/the-history-of-autism/. Accessed on August 02, 2022.

Parsons, S., Yuill, N., Good, J., & Brosnan, M. (2020). 'Whose agenda? Who knows best? Whose voice?' Co-creating a technology research roadmap with autism stakeholders. *Disability & Society*, *35*(2), 201–234.

Peca, A., Coeckelbergh, M., Simut, R., Costescu, C., Pintea, S., David, D., & Vanderborght, B. (2016). Robot enhanced therapy for children with autism disorders: Measuring ethical acceptability. *IEEE Technology and Society Magazine*, *35*(2), 54–66.

Pennisi, P., Tonacci, A., Tartarisco, G., Billeci, L., Ruta, L., Gangemi, S., & Pioggia, G. (2016). Autism and social robotics: A systematic review. *Autism Research*, *9*(2), 165–183.

Phase 2. (2015). National Autism Center at May Institute. Retrieved from https://nationalautismcenter.org/national-standards-project/phase-2/. Accessed on July 06, 2022.

Pryweller, J. R., Schauder, K. B., Anderson, A. W., Heacock, J. L., Foss-Feig, J. H., Newsom, C. R., … Casciofh, C. J. (2014). White matter correlates of sensory processing in autism spectrum disorders. *NeuroImage: Clinical*, *6*, 379–387.

Pulsiri, N., & Vatananan-Thesenvitz, R. (2018) A Systematic literature review of dynamic capabilities, strategic foresight and organizational learning. In *2018 Portland International Conference on Management of Engineering and Technology (PICMET)* (pp. 1–9).

Pulsiri, N., Vatananan-Thesenvitz, R., Tantipisitkul, K., Aung, T. H., Schaller, A.-A., Schaller, A.-M., … Shannon, R. (2019). Achieving Sustainable Development Goals for people with disabilities through digital technologies. In *2019 Portland international conference on management of engineering and technology (PICMET)* (pp. 1–10).

Rabbitt, S. M., Kazdin, A. E., & Scassellati, B. (2015). Integrating socially assistive robotics into mental healthcare interventions: Applications and recommendations for expanded use. *Clinical Psychology Review*, *35*, 35–46.

Rakhymbayeva, N., Amirova, A., & Sandygulova, A. (2021). A long-term engagement with a social robot for autism therapy. *Frontiers in Robotics and AI*, *8*, 180.

Rao, M., & Gershon, M. D. (2016). The bowel and beyond: The enteric nervous system in neurological disorders. *Nature Reviews Gastroenterology & Hepatology*, *13*(9), 517–528.

Rapin, I., & Tuchman, R. F. (2008). Autism: Definition, neurobiology, screening, diagnosis. *Pediatric Clinics of North America*, *55*(5), 1129–1146.

Rice, C. (2013). *Encyclopedia of autism spectrum disorders* (Volkmar F. Editor). New York: Springer.

Richardson, K. (2018). *Challenging sociality: An anthropology of robots, autism, and attachment*. (Online). Retrieved from https://books.google.com/books?hl=en&lr=&id=DqNiDwAAQBAJ&oi=fnd&pg=PR7&dq=neurodiversity+teaching+%22computer+science%22&ots=Df3VnLxgHp&sig=uEikeyY1ogFH0kgl3FOFUsuG1iA

Ricks, D. J., & Colton, M. B. (2010, June). Trends and considerations in robot-assisted autism therapy. *Proceedings of IEEE International Conference on Robotics and Automation* (pp. 4354–4359). doi: 10.1109/ROBOT.2010.5509327

Robins, B., Dautenhahn, K., Te Boekhorst, R., & Billard, A. (2004). Effects of repeated exposure to a humanoid robot on children with autism. In S. Keates, J. Clarkson, P. Langdon & P. Robinson (Eds.), *Designing a more inclusive world* (pp. 225–236). London: Springer. https://doi.org/10.1007/978-0-85729-372-5_23

Robins, B., Dautenhahn, K., Te Boekhorst, R., & Billard, A. (2005). Robotic assistants in therapy and education of children with autism: Can a small humanoid robot help encourage social interaction skills?. *Universal Access in the Information Society*, *4*(2), 105–120.

Robins, B., Dickerson, P., Stribling, P., & Dautenhahn, K. (2004). Robot-mediated joint attention in children with autism: A case study in robot-human interaction. *Interaction Studies*, *5*(2), 161–198. doi: 10.1075/is.5.2.02rob

Rosenwasser, B., & Axelrod, S. (2001). The contributions of applied behavior analysis to the education of people with autism. *Behavior Modification*, *25*(5), 671–677.

Rudovic, O., Lee, J., Mascarell-Maricic, L., Schuller, B. W., & Picard, R. W. (2017). Measuring engagement in robot-assisted autism therapy: A cross-cultural study. *Frontiers in Robotics and AI*, *4*, 36.

Rutter, M. (2005). Aetiology of autism: Findings and questions. *Journal of Intellectual Disability Research*, *49*(4), 231–238.

Rutter, M., Bailey, A., & Lord, C. (2003). *The social communication questionnaire: Manual.* Western Psychological Services.

Snow, A. (2013). Social Communication Questionnaire. In F. R. Volkmar (Eds.), *Encyclopedia of Autism Spectrum Disorders.* New York, NY: Springer. https://doi.org/10.1007/978-1-4419-1698-3_1651

Rutter, M., Le Couteur, A., Lord, C. (2003). Autism diagnostic interview-revised. *Western Psychological Services Reviews in Los Angeles, CA*, *29*(2003), 30.

Salam, H., Celiktutan, O., Hupont, I., Gunes, H., & Chetouani, M. (2016). Fully automatic analysis of engagement and its relationship to personality in human–robot interactions. *IEEE Access*, *5*, 705–721.

Sanders, S. J., He, X., Jeremy Willsey, A., Gulhan Ercan-Sencicek, A., Samocha, K. E., Ercument Cicek, A., … State, M. W. (2015). Insights into autism spectrum disorder genomic architecture and biology from 71 risk loci. *Neuron*, *87*(6), 1215–1233.

Scassellati, B. (2005). Quantitative metrics of social response for autism diagnosis. In *ROMAN 2005. IEEE international workshop on robot and human interactive communication* (pp. 585–590).

Scassellati, B., Admoni, H., & Matarić, M. (2012). Robots for use in autism research. *Annual Review of Biomedical Engineering*, *14*, 275–294.

Scassellati, B., Boccanfuso, L., Huang, C.-M., Mademtzi, M., Qin, M., Salomons, N., … Shic, F. (2018). Improving social skills in children with ASD using a long-term, in-home social robot. *Science Robotics*, *3*(21), 1–10. doi: 10.1126/scirobotics.aat7544.

Schaller, A.-A., Vatananan-Thesenvitz, R., & Stefania, M. (2018). Business model innovation roadmapping: A structured approach to a new business model. In *2018 Portland International Conference on Management of Engineering and Technology (PICMET)* (pp. 1–9).

Schmidt, M., Newbutt, N., Schmidt, C., & Glaser, N. (2021). A process-model for minimizing adverse effects when using head mounted display-based virtual reality for individuals with autism. *Frontiers in Virtual Reality*, 2, 13.

Schopler, E., Reichler, R. J., & Renner, B. R. (1988). *The Childhood Autism Rating Scale.* Los Angeles, CA: Western Psychological Services.

Science Digital. (2022). Assistive Technologies for People with Disability: Education – Science Digital @ UNGA 75. Retrieved from http://

sciencedigitalunga75.com/events/assistive-technologies/. Accessed on March 23, 2022.

Seltzer, M. M., Shattuck, P., Abbeduto, L., & Greenberg, J. S. (2004). Trajectory of development in adolescents and adults with autism. *Mental Retardation and Developmental Disabilities Research Reviews*, *10*(4), 234–247.

Shattuck, P. T. (2006). The contribution of diagnostic substitution to the growing administrative prevalence of autism in US special education. *Pediatrics*, *117*(4), 1028–1037.

Shukla, J., Cristiano, J., Amela, D., Anguera, L., Vergés-Llahí, J., & Puig, D. (2015). A case study of robot interaction among individuals with profound and multiple learning disabilities. In *International conference on social robotics* (pp. 613–622).

Simpson, R. L., de Boer-Ott, S. R., & Smith-Myles, B. (2003). Inclusion of learners with autism spectrum disorders in general education settings. *Topics in Language Disorders*, *23*(2), 116–133.

Smith, T., & Iadarola, S. (2015). Evidence base update for autism spectrum disorder. *Journal of Clinical Child & Adolescent Psychology*, *44*(6), 897–922.

So, W.-C., Wong, M.-Y., Cabibihan, J.-J., Lam, C.-Y., Chan, R.-Y., & Qian, H.-H. (2016). Using robot animation to promote gestural skills in children with autism spectrum disorders. *Journal of Computer Assisted Learning*, *32*(6), 632–646.

So, W.-C., Wong, M. K.-Y., Lui, M., & Yip, V. (2015). The development of co-speech gesture and its semantic integration with speech in 6-to 12-year-old children with autism spectrum disorders. *Autism*, *19*(8), 956–968.

Spiel, K., Brulé, E., Frauenberger, C., Bailly, G., & Fitzpatrick, G. (2018). Micro-ethics for participatory design with marginalised children. In *Proceedings of the 15th participatory design conference: Full Papers-Volume 1* (pp. 1–12).

Szymona, B., Maciejewski, M., Karpiński, R., Jonak, K., Radzikowska-Büchner, E., Niderla, K., & Prokopiak, A. (2021). Robot-Assisted Autism Therapy (RAAT). Criteria and types of experiments using anthropomorphic and zoomorphic robots. Review of the research. *Sensors*, *21*(11), 3720.

The Guardian. (2022). How robots are helping children with autism | Health & wellbeing | The Guardian. Retrieved from https://www.

theguardian.com/lifeandstyle/2015/feb/01/how-robots-helping-children-with-autism. Accessed on July 08, 2022.

Thill, S., Pop, C. A., Belpaeme, T., Ziemke, T., & Vanderborght, B. (2012). Robot-assisted therapy for autism spectrum disorders with (partially) autonomous control: Challenges and outlook. *Paladyn*, *3*(4), 209–217.

Tolksdorf, N. F., & Rohlfing, K. J. (2020). Parents' views on using social robots for language learning. In *2020 29th IEEE international conference on robot and human interactive communication (RO-MAN)* (pp. 634–640).

Tribune. (2022). 400k Pakistani children suffer from autism. Retrieved from https://tribune.com.pk/story/2292799/400k-pakistani-children-suffer-from-autism. Accessed on February 22, 2022.

U. N. G. Assembly. (2015). *Transforming our world: The 2030 agenda for sustainable development*, 21 October 2015.

Vahabzadeh, A., Keshav, N. U., Abdus-Sabur, R., Huey, K., Liu, R., & Sahin, N. T. (2018). Improved socio-emotional and behavioral functioning in students with autism following school-based smartglasses intervention: Multi-stage feasibility and controlled efficacy study. *Behavioral Sciences (Basel, Switzerland)*, *8*(10), 85.

Valadão, C. T., Goulart, C., Rivera, H., Caldeira, E., Filho, T. F. B., Frizera-Neto, A., & Carelli, R. (2016). Analysis of the use of a robot to improve social skills in children with autism spectrum disorder. *Research on Biomedical Engineering*, *32*, 161–175.

Vohr, B. R., Davis, E. P., Wanke, C. A., & Krebs, N. F. (2017). Neurodevelopment: The impact of nutrition and inflammation during preconception and pregnancy in low-resource settings. *Pediatrics*, *139*(Supplement 1), S38–S49.

Volkmar, F. R., State, M., & Klin, A. (2009). Autism and autism spectrum disorders: Diagnostic issues for the coming decade. *Journal of Child Psychology and Psychiatry*, *50*(1–2), 108–115.

Wasilewska, J., & Klukowski, M. (2015). Gastrointestinal symptoms and autism spectrum disorder: Links and risks – A possible new overlap syndrome. *Pediatric Health, Medicine and Therapeutics*, *6*, 153.

Wilbarger, J., Gunnar, M., Schneider, M., & Pollak, S. (2010). Sensory processing in internationally adopted, post-institutionalized children. *Journal of Child Psychology and Psychiatry*, *51*(10), 1105–1114.

Wilkinson, K. M., Light, J., & Drager, K. (2012, September). Considerations for the composition of visual scene displays: Potential contributions of information from visual and cognitive sciences (Forum Note). *Augmentative and Alternative Communication, 28*(3), 137. doi: 10.3109/07434618.2012.704522

Williams, R. M., & Gilbert, J. E. (2020). Perseverations of the academy: A survey of wearable technologies applied to autism intervention. *International Journal of Human-Computer Studies, 143*, 102485.

Wilson, J., & Rosenberg, D. (1988). Rapid prototyping for user interface design. In M. Helander (Ed.), *Handbook of human-computer interaction* (pp. 859–875). Amsterdam: North-Holland.. Retrieved from https://www.scirp.org/(S(351jmbntvnsjt1aadkposzje))/reference/ReferencesPapers.aspx?ReferenceID=1986656. Accessed on February 23, 2022.

Wood, L. J., Zaraki, A., Robins, B., & Dautenhahn, K. (2021). Developing kaspar: A humanoid robot for children with autism. *International Journal of Social Robotics, 13*, 491–508.

World Health Organization (WHO). (2007). *International classification of functioning, disability, and health: Children & youth version: ICF-CY*. World Health Organization.

World Health Organization (WHO). (2022). Autism spectrum disorders. Retrieved from https://www.who.int/news-room/fact-sheets/detail/autism-spectrum-disorders. Accessed on February 22, 2022.

Yang, S., & Zhang, J. (2021, September). Book Review: A computational view of autism: Using virtual reality technologies in autism intervention. *Frontiers in Psychology, 0*, 4166. doi: 10.3389/FPSYG.2021.722672

Zervogianni, V., Fletcher-Watson, S., Herrera, G., Goodwin, M., Pérez-Fuster, P., Brosnan, M., & Grynszpan, O. (2020). A framework of evidence-based practice for digital support, co-developed with and for the autism community. *Autism, 24*(6), 1411–1422.

Zhang, Y., Song, W., Tan, Z., Wang, Y., Lam, C. M., Hoi, S. P., … Yi, L. (2019). Theory of Robot Mind: False belief attribution to social robots in children with and without autism. *Frontiers in Psychology, 10*, 1732.

Zhang, Y., Song, W., Tan, Z., Zhu, H., Wang, Y., Lam, C. M., … Yi, L. (2019). Could social robots facilitate children with autism spectrum disorders in learning distrust and deception? *Computers in Human Behavior, 98*, 140–149.

INDEX

Printed and bound by CPI Group (UK) Ltd, Croydon, CR0 4YY

13/09/2026

14961061-0004